SEXUAL RADIANCE

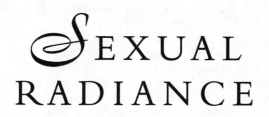

SEXUAL
RADIANCE

—

A 21-Day Program
for
Vitality and Sensuality

Susan Taylor, Ph.D.

THREE RIVERS PRESS
New York

This book is not intended to substitute for consultation with a qualified medical practitioner. The 21-day program of breathwork, nutrition, and exercise is presented solely for informational and educational purposes and not as medical advice. The author recommends consultation with a medical practitioner before beginning any part of the program.

The author or her agents will not accept responsibility for injury, loss, or damage occasioned to any person acting or refraining from action as a result of material in this book, whether or not such injury, loss, or damage is due in any way to any negligent act or omission, breach of duty, or default on the part of the author or her agents.

For the sake of privacy, the names of the patients whose stories are told in this book and personal details that might identify them have been changed.

Copyright © 1998 by Susan Taylor, Ph.D.

Published by Three Rivers Press,
201 East 50th Street, New York, New York 10022.
Member of the Crown Publishing Group.

Originally published in hardcover by Harmony Books, 1998.

Random House, Inc. New York, Toronto, London, Sydney, Auckland
www.randomhouse.com

Three Rivers Press is a registered trademark of Random House, Inc.

Printed in the United States of America

Design by Susan Hood
Illustrations by Jennifer Harper

Library of Congress Cataloging-in-Publication Data
Taylor, Susan, Ph.D.
Sexual radiance : a 21-day program for vitality and sensuality /
Susan Taylor. Includes index. (alk. paper)
1. Sex—Health aspects.   2. Sexual attraction—Health aspects.
3. Women—Health and hygiene.   4. Metabolism.   I. Title.
HQ23.T38   1998
613.9'54—dc21   98-15209

ISBN 0-609-80481-2

10 9 8 7 6 5 4 3 2 1

First Paperback Edition

TO MY SPIRITUAL MASTER, WHO HAS GIVEN ME
UNCONDITIONAL LOVE AND SHOWED ME THE
RAREST COMPASSION ONE COULD EVER KNOW.
WITH DEEPEST GRATITUDE, I DEDICATE MY
LIFE'S WORK TO HIM.

$\mathscr{A}$CKNOWLEDGMENTS

Writing this book has been a lifelong dream and one that has changed my life. I could not have accomplished it without the support, guidance, and influence of many people.

I am so very grateful to the following people, who have been instrumental in providing the structure with which this book has manifested.

My deepest gratitude to Shaye Areheart for her dedication, support, and acceptance, without which this new edition of the book would not exist. Leslie Meredith, who always believed in this book. Dina Siciliano for her excellent assistance in a myriad of ways. Kate Reid for her extra publicity efforts. Laura Wood for her original editorial work, and the Harmony production staff who made this project possible.

Thanks also to Nancy Kahan, my publicist, for her intuition and support. Barb Shultz and Jennie Kramer, who brought me to my literary agent. Dick Marek, for his guidance and expertise in bringing the level of writing to mastery. Special thanks to my literary agent, Janis Vallely, who intuitively understood this material from our first meeting and supported me throughout this project. Jennifer Harper, for her considerable talent in preparing the illustrations.

My deepest gratitude to my friend Phil Nuernberger, who introduced me to the tradition twenty years ago. I am grateful for his review of the manuscript and his counsel and support. I am deeply grateful to Rose Marie Raccioppi for opening an inner vision that allowed me to read fully for the first time. Special thanks to my friend and science mentor, Dr. Henri Brunengraber, who trained me to be a scientist through many years of patience and compassion. I am also indebted to my clients, who allowed me to share in their growth process. If they have received half as much from me as I have from them, I would be more than happy.

And thanks to my parents for their love, wisdom, and encouragement, which have supported me on my life's journey. And to my siblings, Andrew, Paul, and Anna, for their highly evolved spirits, which exhibit unconditional love.

I wish to acknowledge finally the enlightened masters who mentor and nourish me, and who remind me how beautiful life really is—for it is they who have given me the privilege of writing this book. Without their guidance, I would have little to say.

CONTENTS

SEXUAL RADIANCE

ℳY SEXUAL ODYSSEY

I was the perfect child. Again and again my father told me so, and my mother—without so high a degree of certainty, it seemed to me—agreed. I didn't complain, I didn't act out, I did what I was told, and I was rewarded for it. What better way for me to secure my parents' love than to be "perfect"?

So I was an obedient child, a model student, the girl who "cleaned up her room and helped her mother," and praise flowed. The pressure was tremendous. I dared not slip.

My family was Catholic, not deeply religious but strict followers of Catholic moral law. My father was a hardworking family man, and remnants of religious training remained in his character. When I was a young child, my father would often read to me from the Bible, and I came to see Jesus as a well-educated Yogi—a man of infinite wisdom, a great teacher, a mentor.

Sex, according to my family, was something one simply did not talk about, let alone do. Like many children of the late 1950s, and even today, I received no sexual education and as a teenager listened with a combination of awe and fear as my girlfriends talked of secret petting sessions and open lust. Still, I was a person born into the "golden penis syndrome," in that my world was to revolve around men. They were to make the decisions and I was to give away part of myself in order to satisfy them. This was an idea that permeated my entire life, including my early sexual life.

It was my brain that gave me my self-esteem, my intellectual prowess, for though I was dyslexic, I realized I was smarter than my friends. They, however, seemed to be having more fun; they were "smarter" in matters of the body. I decided I was a frump, and dressed accordingly in baggy clothes, gorged on ice cream and cookies, did not menstruate until I was seventeen, had a series of urinary tract infections, and avoided boys. I was perfect, all right: a perfect student and a perfect daughter—but a failure as a girl.

Despite my sexual education (or lack of it), it did not seem right to wait until I got married to have sex, so I came up with my own rule: I would not have intercourse with anyone until it was entirely my decision (not the boy's) to do so, and that decision would be predicated on my feeling that the boy and I shared a spiritual as well as a physical attraction.

I waited until my freshman year at college. My first lover was an older man without much sexual expertise. I enjoyed the act, having had no idea that there was more to sex than spasms, and enjoyed our after-sex sessions when we would sit together and share a quart of ice cream. Being Catholic, I was taught that the first guy you slept with was the man you married, but he called me stupid one day, and I (luckily!) dropped whatever thoughts of marriage I might have had. Later he told me he had insulted me because he was afraid I would leave him "to become a doctor," but at the time I believed he really meant it, and so took up with an older man who thought I was "a genius" and encouraged me to read.

He was as bad at sex as I was at reading, so we taught each other. I showed him how to breathe during sex (I knew how instinctively; I only understood why breath is so important and made it part of my formal program years later). He showed me that I could learn from reading as well as life—without that knowledge I could not have formulated my regimen or written this book. He was a mentor, but while I was still with him, I fell in love with a different man.

His name was Gary. He was a medical student and rock musician; he liked drugs and loved sex. Still the "perfect" girl, I supported him through his residency by taking a job as a teacher of exercise and yoga, all the while completing graduate work at Columbia University. I rarely shared his drugs—even then I generally steered clear of poison—but his ardor, his passion, and his enjoyment in both the physical and spiritual components of lovemaking awakened me to the possibilities of sex, and for the first time I knew what it meant to be a sexual woman.

He told me I was beautiful and I tried to make myself *more* beautiful. I lost weight, wore miniskirts and short-sleeved blouses, and, most important, felt inside myself a vitality, an energy, a joy in life, a pleasure at being me.

Eventually Gary and I broke up. I had told him I could not go on with him if he continued to take drugs, but he preferred drugs—and another woman.

I went wild with rage and was consumed by depression; the two go hand in hand. I took a revenge lover but could not have an orgasm. My weight went from 108 to 148 pounds, for I substituted nighttime food for nighttime sex. The urinary tract infections of my adolescence returned. I was literally *pissed off.* Doctors told me my urethra was out of line, that my ovaries were tilted. I wore bulky sweaters and shapeless jeans. I felt no sexual desire. I found men threatening. I wanted only to escape.

I went back to my childhood strengths, my intellect and an almost uncanny intuition, and accepted a scholarship to Case Western Reserve University in Cleveland, where I began working toward a Ph.D. in human nutrition. Cleveland took me as far as possible from my former life.

I planned to write my doctoral thesis on "Nutritional Aspects of Taekwondo Athletes," Taekwondo being a martial arts Olympic sport, and spent a good deal of time at the Olympic center in Colorado Springs, Colorado, watching with the eyes of a dumpy woman thirty pounds overweight the training of some of the most beautiful bodies in the world.

I knew there was something seriously out of balance. I knew the changes in my body did not have to happen, that depression and rage did not have to dominate my life, but I did not know what to do about it. Then one day a doctor told me that my urinary tract infection was "normal," that other female disorders such as candida were "normal," that depression was "normal," that *disease* was "normal."

Candida? his attitude suggested. Stick in a monostad suppository.

Urinary tract infection? Take an antibiotic.

Depression? There's a wonderful new drug called Prozac.

I listened to him with increasing horror, but when I left I knew I had found my life's work.

I knew from my yoga teaching, from my research in nutrition at Case, from my gut, and from the remembered experience of my own energy and "aliveness" when I was with Gary that "normal" meant vitality, self-assurance, joy, health, sex, pleasure, love. Disease was *ab*normal, depression was *ab*normal, stress was something we imposed on ourselves *that did not have to be!* I knew from my own fascination with the healthy body and my unalterable determination to be master of myself that what my doctor had told me was plain loony.

No doctor could cure me, I knew. The only person who could restore my sexuality, my vitality, my sense of well-being was me.

And if I could bring radiance back into my life, I could bring it into the lives of others.

———

After two years of study and having finished my Ph.D. qualifiers, my department chairman at Case was replaced by a nutritional biochemist who stressed laboratory research over fieldwork, and I switched my thesis topic to the effect of starvation—deprivation of glucose—on tumors. I worked with rats, and I found that when a body is put under metabolic stress, it creates metabolic imbalances; this was a revelation to me, and it altered my thinking about the effects of different foods on the body. I also worked on the biochemical and physiological effects of carbohydrates, fats, and proteins on metabolism during normal bodily states as well as during states of stress, and was able even then to formulate the essential core of my present program.

My weight was still up, so I tried a grapefruit diet. It failed. I tried the water diet. Useless. I tried fasting—for as long as twenty-four days I ingested nothing but water and fresh juices—and of course I lost weight, but I put it back on as soon as I ended the diet, and I felt no better for it. An overnight fast is part of my program, but it has more to do with the timing of what you ingest than the weight you'll lose because of it.

I realized then that there was no magic formula, no miracle regimen that would enable me to lose weight permanently and regain my lost vitality, but that the way to radiant health had to do with regulating the metabolic process. If I could burn the food I ate more quickly, transforming it into energy, I would literally become "hot," not only as a sexual metaphor but biochemically as well.

For ten years, I had been teaching exercise and breathing to women, noting how much better they felt and livelier they seemed when they followed a regular program. Because yoga was fundamental to my classes, I continued to read the Vedic texts, which had been introduced to me by an Indian Tantric teacher and spiritual master, who demonstrated techniques from the East I was able to apply to my life in the West. Because of him, I decided to devote myself to helping others.

The Vedic texts taught me the existence of the seven chakras, disparate energy systems located throughout the body that govern all facets of human life: fear, sexuality, power, love, creativity, intuition, and knowledge. (Acupuncture meridians are based on a similar concept.)

Energy systems, I thought. Precisely the subject that was becoming more and more fascinating to me. Food, exercise, breathing, all affecting metabolism. Metabolism is the *creation* of energy, and now I knew there were specific locations in the body that could be directly influenced by it.

It was all coming together. I had already been maintaining a steady regimen of breathing and exercise. Now I added a twenty-one-day diet, breathing, and exercise plan that regulated metabolism, and quickly found out *when* to eat as well as *what* to eat. I learned about herbs, about flower extracts, about body temperature.

Almost without my recognizing it, I became rejuvenated. I began to lose weight. I was able to love my body and in so doing love myself. My depression lifted. I regained my sexual appetite and—no coincidence!—met David.

Once, right after we had made love, he looked at me with enormous tenderness and joy. I smiled back at him, seeing and sharing his pleasure.

"You look radiant," he said.

———

After I received my Ph.D., I was offered postdoc positions at Berkeley and Harvard, but I turned them down. From now on, I decided, I would work with my own clients, with people who needed the kind of discovery or rediscovery of their sexual selves that I had experienced. My private practice focuses on teaching people that they have the power to heal themselves. My work is holistic, which means I use a regimen that treats the entire person and the cause of a given condition as opposed to just the system. People don't come to me at first specifically for sexual therapy (almost always it's for stress-related issues), but they come without knowing what it means to be vital, and "vital" means being sexually radiant. Over the last four years, hundreds of women, from TV personalities to corporate executives to housewives, have benefited from my ministrations.

If hundreds, why not thousands? I asked myself. And so I began to write this book.

Part I

—

THE METABOLIC CONNECTION

Chapter 1

THE MYSTERY OF SEXUAL RADIANCE

Years ago, we called it "It," that undefinable quality that some women have and others don't. Later we called it sex appeal. Some women were born with it, we felt. They could just naturally turn guys on.

Women who had it didn't have to be physically attractive; men would flock to them anyway. At parties they were surrounded, whereas other women stood virtually alone, having to seek out companionship rather than letting it come to them. Often these women had a succession of lovers. In other cases, they married the "best catch," even if far more beautiful women had pursued him.

Sex appeal—that certain something—was a mysterious quality, one we couldn't comprehend. Perhaps it was genetic, like blue eyes. Surely it didn't have to do with overt sexual provocativeness; indeed, many of the sexiest girls were happily married and seemingly oblivious of their ability to attract. Their dresses were no shorter or more revealing; they did not parade around in Lycra or advertise their breasts with push-up bras. Yet there the men were—there the men and *women* were—though we were just as pretty, just as smart, and had just as much to contribute.

I know now why women are sexy: They have sexual radiance. And I don't believe it's genetic, I don't believe that "either you have it or you don't," I don't believe that luck has anything to do with it. Sexual radiance is a quality innate in all women. If you don't have it now, you can evoke it; if you've lost it, you can bring it back.

It is not at all mysterious, though it may seem so. Follow my program, and you'll see it transform your life.

———

When I first met her, Diana didn't have it.

She was depressed, but antidepressants did little good for her. She suffered from a variety of severe stomach ailments (indigestion, reflux, and gas) and occasional urinary tract infections, but no prescribed medicine could cure them. Although married for only two years (she was thirty-two), she had lost interest in sex. "I endure it," she told me, "because I adore my husband and want him to be happy. But it's getting more and more difficult. When we make love, I get so tense I want to bolt. There's no pleasure in it. Yet when we were first married, I couldn't get enough!"

Diana was pretty, with a figure going toward fat but not yet there, and long black hair swept up into a ponytail. She was pale and there was such pain in her eyes that my heart ached at the sight of it. Her physician had recommended me, she said. He had heard I could do "wonders" with female ailments. "He hasn't really been able to find anything medically wrong with me," she sighed, as though this was something to be ashamed of. "But I'm always tired, and I don't seem to be able to laugh anymore."

"Tell me about yourself," I said. "Do you work?"

"For an advertising agency. Account executive. High stress, good pay."

"Wining and dining of clients?"

"All the time."

"Late meals?"

"They can last past ten."

"Yet you're only a little overweight."

"I don't eat lunch," she explained, as though revealing a secret.

I could barely keep from smiling. This case, I thought, was going to be a (metaphorical) piece of cake.

"Describe your diet," I said. "Leafy greens?"

She looked at me, puzzled. "What are they?"

I was not surprised she didn't know; many people don't. "Green vegetables. Salads, spinach."

She hesitated. "I suppose so. There's always a vegetable with the main course."

"Desserts?"

"Sometimes. I try to stay away from them, but I love sweets."

"And wine?"

"A glass or two." She shrugged. "I really don't see what this all has to do with sex."

"You will," I said. "Coffee?"

"I'd love a cup."

I laughed. "I don't mean here. Do you drink coffee at night?"

"Decaf. But I drink the strong stuff in the morning."

"I see. Do you exercise?"

"No regular program. But I walk *everywhere.*"

"Which is more important," I asked, "your sex life or those client dinners?"

"My sex life!" she blurted. "But I couldn't give up—"

"You don't have to give them up. You have to *change* them."

"Change them how?"

"By eating as little as possible at night. And maybe by changing the dinners to lunches, or at least making them earlier in the evenings. Would that be possible?"

"I suppose so. In fact, most of my clients would probably welcome it."

"At lunch," I told her, "you can eat as much as you want. Sweets, too, though you probably won't crave them after a while."

She was obviously astonished. "I don't get it," she said. "What's the difference whether you eat a lot at lunch or at supper?"

Diana would need more than just a change of diet, I knew. I would prescribe supplements as well, plus teach her how to breathe and how to move. But her question was familiar: It had been asked by dozens of my clients, enough so I became aware of how little knowledge women have about what affects their sexuality.

"Have you ever heard of metabolism?" I asked.

"I've *heard* of it, but I'm not sure . . ."

I explained.

Three months later, Diana came in for what was to be the last of her biweekly visits. There was a bounce to her walk and she was smiling, but there were dark circles under her eyes.

"You look tired," I said.

"I'm exhausted." She was grinning.

"Late client meeting?"

She blushed. "Late *husband* meeting. We made love four times last night. Neither of us could stop."

––––––

My clients arrive at my office in generally poor health. There is often nothing overtly wrong with them, yet their symptoms include fatigue, depression, weight gain, stress. All of them report sexual dysfunction: lack of desire, vaginal dryness, apathy. *And all of them can be helped!*

They are women who have gone too long without a proper regimen for health, without knowing that their lives could be easier, happier, more youthful, more vital, more *radiant,* if they only found the key to metabolic energy through my system of nutrition, movement, and breathing technique.

Just walking along the street, you'll be able to differentiate between the vital women and the sad sacks. One walks with her upper torso bent forward and pelvis back, as though she's afraid to expose her sexual vulnerability. Another wears clothes that are a tent big enough for several people. A third strides purposefully, shoulders back, pelvis out. Her hair falls luxuriantly around her shoulders; her clothes are form-fitting but not blatantly so. She doesn't need high heels or dramatic cleavage to be the sexiest woman on the street.

You can become more like the third woman. No matter how old you are or what your unique physical characteristics are, you can achieve a more balanced metabolism and a more energetic self. There is nothing in my program that's complicated or unpleasant. The nutritional program contains a variety of foods, and you won't go hungry (except at night, but you'll get used to it); the movements involve no special machinery (neither Exercycles nor NordicTracks, though both have their benefits); the breathing, once practiced, will become as natural as, well, *breathing,* and you won't have to think about it again.

Proper nutrition, movement, and breathing are all factors in maximizing your metabolic potential, and sexual radiance is the result, an inner energetic vitality that shines through your mind and your body, that makes you a sexual being even when sexual intercourse is the furthest thing from your mind. The sexually radiant woman has sparkling eyes, walks with a spring to her step, takes pleasure in the physical world and the world of ideas, is adventurous, open to experience, self-confident—and loves to make love.

Of course there will still be moments when you feel down, lethargic, unattractive, stressed; I'm a nutritional biochemist, not a miracle worker. Life can and will bring heartache regardless of my program. But when that happens you'll regain equilibrium faster, feel less stressed sooner, come back to your sexiness and vitality in less time if you follow my program. It's as simple as understanding your metabolism—and learning ways to invigorate it.

————

Here is my definition of sexual radiance and the theory of metabolic vitality that is the centerpiece of my program.

Female sexuality is the sum total of our spirituality, our ability to nurture, our ability to *be* nurtured, the expression of our most profound feelings, and our erotic impulse. All of these elements come together to form our true essence, which resides in our deepest selves. It allows us emotional and physical expression. It accounts for our creativity, our passion, our moods, our tears, and our laughter.

Sexual radiance is the ability to experience our true selves most fully, and to transmit that sense of inner completeness to our lovers, our families, and our friends. When we feel whole and intact, we draw others to us like a magnet, and in the process our biochemical selves become better equipped to lessen the effects of many "women's problems," such as PMS, menopause, fibroids, and urinary tract infections. We feel strong and open to possibilities, open to intimacy.

Sexual radiance is health and is as essential to living as oxygen.

———

Since the basis for sexual radiance is metabolism, and metabolism is a biochemical process, we can learn how to adjust it, fine-tune it, bring it to life from its dormancy, and make it give off heat.

A chemist would define metabolism as combustion, the act of creating fire. Fire has one universal purpose, to transform matter into energy, and that is precisely what metabolism does. The more efficient our metabolic process is, the more energetic we feel. The more energetic we feel, the greater our sexual radiance. It's as simple as that.

When our metabolism is up and running, our bodies automatically "manufacture" sexual energy. By learning to increase metabolic efficiency, we can prolong the "normal" course of sexual aging and increase our vitality, our years of ideal health.

Our metabolism is influenced by biochemical processes, which in turn are regulated by enzymatic reactions, hormonal fluctuations, and biochemical components like essential fatty acids and amino acids. These biomedical processes are directly affected and "fed" by our nutrition, exercise, and breathing. Thus the more effectively we learn to eat, move, and breathe, the more we can directly or indirectly trigger our metabolism to function at its maximum strength. As a simple example, if you eat a high-fat, high-sugar lunch, the body must divert all its energy to processing the sugar and fat. The result will be "metabolic fatigue," and you'll be hard pressed to be creative, think clearly, work efficiently—or have good sex.

Our diet, movement, and breath affect our metabolism on a cellular level by way of blood flow to the heart and lungs. Our bloodstream brings nutrient-rich blood to all the organic systems in the body, including the brain, which acts as our internal computer, governing our emotions and our physical activities, and the liver, which serves as our metabolic hotel, doing the housecleaning throughout our system by removing toxins from the food we eat and the air we breathe. Proper nutrition, movement, and breathing cuts down on the work the liver has to do and frees the brain to be its most efficient. Sexual vitality is one of the results.

————

While much of the theory of sexual radiance may be new to the West, it has been long known in the East. The reason Eastern sexual practice concentrates on multiple orgasms for women and delayed ejaculation for men is that nature has designed women in such a way that sexual vitality does not deplete their vital resources, but rather enhances them—the opposite of men—due to the fact that women must maintain their ability to bear, nourish, and protect their offspring. That's good luck for us.

Good metabolism determines good sexual vitality, and good sexual vitality means good health. I will show you how to maintain proper metabolism so that you will be subject to fewer illnesses, your chances of contracting a disease will lessen, and your aging process will slow. You can run marathons and diet until you're a beanpole, but unless you learn to work with your own individual metabolic process, you will fall subject to a range of ordinary ailments, both transient and long term, that could have easily been avoided.

In general, suppressed sexual energy can be a causative factor in disease, which is why my program is essential for anyone over fifty. Moreover, many diseases are based upon or involve the wrong use of sexual energy—including diseases of the mind, since many psychological disorders are based on an inability to form the right relationships with others and with the self. That is why my program is essential for the young as well, for unless you learn to "manufacture" sexual energy—that is, make sure your metabolism is working smoothly, that it burns fuel at neither too high nor too low a rate—your health is in jeopardy whether you are twenty-five or sixty-five.

Maintenance of the proper metabolism can be enhanced by herbs that energize the reproductive system and stimulate and promote sexual vitality. These herbs have been prescribed in the East for ages but are now also available in the West, and I'll specify them in the section on diet and nutrition, along with flower essences, invaluable tools for enhancing the spiritual and emotional components of sexuality and health.

———

In the West, where too often sex is simply intercourse divorced from emotion, creativity, and spirituality—a mechanical act for the purposes of reproduction or a transient pleasure—we consider it the province of the young. We assume that our sexual power will be depleted as we age, that postmenopausal women are sexually "worthless" since they can no longer reproduce, and that in time men will no longer be able to "get it up" or want to.

That is why our culture, in its attitudes, popular literature, movies, and TV, and particularly in its advertising, promotes the idea that we must maintain youth at all costs (the women in ads for, say, life insurance, dentures, and panty shields look, or are made to look, far younger than the "real" women who are the consumers of these products). And it's also why older people are so prone to heart ailments, and ovarian and prostate cancer, diseases far less common in the East, where sexuality is believed to be just as vital in later life as in youth, and where sexual attractiveness is based not on looks but on radiance.

Sexual radiance can be a lifelong gift you give to yourself. I have a friend whose widowed mother remarried at the age of eighty! "I couldn't keep my hands off her," her new, eighty-two-year-old husband explained to me. "There's just something about her. . . ."

His voice trailed off because he couldn't find the words to explain what made her so desirable. But I can: sexual radiance.

———

In the following chapters, I'm going to be specific about just what foods to eat, what exercises to do, what breathing techniques to use to best speed up the metabolic process. I will end with a three-week program devised to bring maximum results in a minimum amount of time, but be warned that if you fall back into sloppy habits, these techniques and the overall program will lose their effect.

Still, exceptions can be made. You'll learn that the bulk of your eating (pun intended) should take place between ten A.M. and two P.M., but if there is a client dinner or an important date with your partner, eat away, but avoid sex that night. If you're new to the program and crave sugar, as I do, by all means eat the cookies, cake, or ice cream you love most, but do it between 10 A.M. and 2 P.M. (By the second or third week, I think you'll find that sugar-laden foods will have lost their allure.) If a specific herb tastes awful to you, skip it. If the leg exercises I prescribe take too much time on workdays, do them over the weekends, but make sure you substitute a different exercise during the week, one you can do in the office. If in moments of stress you don't always breathe from your diaphragm, go on breathing anyway!

My program is designed for all women, but I recognize that each woman is different, and that what works for one will not—because of circumstances, body characteristics, schedule, personality, lifestyle, and so on—work as well for another, so some fine-tuning may be called for. I *hate* diet books that promise success for everyone thanks to the food pyramid or the ingestion of a specific food group (just fruit, say, or protein-rich foods). I believe your own body should dictate what exercises you perform, so long as you get *enough* exercise to keep your metabolism in full gear. The exercises in my program are specifically designed to stimulate sexual vitality. And while I practice meditation and breathing for an hour every day and recommend it highly, it may not be right for everyone. As long as you learn to breathe so that good breathing becomes natural to you, meditation is not essential—but I encourage you to give it a try.

————

Sexual radiance only *seems* mysterious. You can solve the mystery and incorporate sexual radiance into your essence. It will *become* your essence. "Something about you has changed," your friends will say. And your sexual partners will find you more attractive; their own sexual appetite will grow as yours does.

My overall program is more important than its specifics, but if you follow it, results are guaranteed. As you start, remember:

- Overeating or eating the wrong foods is like putting wet wood on a fire. And metabolic fire is what gives us sexual radiance.
- Eating processed, nonorganic, or canned foods is like using low-test gasoline when your car needs premium.
- It is better to do half my program correctly than to do it all incorrectly. (But it's far better to do it *all* correctly.)

- When cells age or become damaged, raw fruits and vegetables—the best sources for vitamins and minerals—will replenish them.
- The best healer of the body is the body itself.
- Caffeine, diet pills, and extended fasting are sure ways to destroy vitality. All will reduce the production of enzymes and hormones, and while you may lose weight temporarily, you'll also be losing *you,* since your body will only feed on itself to get the nourishment it needs.
- Abdominal and diaphragmatic breathing takes energy from the air and pumps it into your lungs, which will then pump it throughout your system.
- Stress adversely affects sex hormones, and proper breathing reduces stress.
- Exercise can cause problems if it creates stress rather than reduces it.
- Both the upper body and lower body should be exercised, for both affect the pelvic and abdominal centers by increasing the flow of enzymes and hormones.
- Your own sexual radiance will elicit radiance in others, women as well as men.
- You don't need a Wonder bra, a miniskirt, bright red lipstick, high heels, or exotic perfumes to seem sexually vital. You need sexual vitality.
- The best of all vitalizing substances is a partner who loves you. And the best way to find one is to be fully receptive and sexually radiant when you meet.

Before we start the program, put a check mark beside each symptom that applies to you.

_____ Fatigue or exhaustion
_____ Lack of sexual desire
_____ Bladder problems
_____ Menstrual problems

____ Hormonal imbalance
____ Take medications
____ Depression
____ Irritability
____ Headaches
____ Digestive problems
____ Low self-esteem
____ Feel overworked
____ Feel emotionally burdened
____ Overweight
____ Underweight
____ Constipation
____ Diarrhea
____ Lack of exercise
____ Breathe from chest
____ Sick more than once a year
____ Difficulty getting up in the morning
____ Insomnia
____ Feel hesitant
____ Feel unattractive
____ Feel shy
____ Feel fear
____ Feel unloved

If you've checked a number of these—or even one—read on!

Chapter 2

ENERGY MODULATION

Sexual intercourse is an exchange of energy. For a man, entering a woman's body—a woman who has the energy to "grow" a child—is a pleasurable privilege, for it enables him to partake of at least a small portion of that energy. From the woman's perspective, when a man ejaculates, his fluid has a great deal of subtle energy, and she partakes of this. The man's energy is dependent on his physical state of health and his mental state of awareness and love, so if he is depressed, or fundamentally uninterested in the woman, she may not be experiencing beneficial energy at all. Because of this energy exchange, women who have many partners are often confused sexually about the men making love to them.

Energy is shared on a biological level through fluid exchange and on a psychic level through the breath and thought process. The vibrations that pulse through one body are felt by the other. Native Americans believe that when a woman makes love, she draws her partner to her through a cord (there is a different cord for each partner), and the partner feeds off this cord. If she has many sexual partners during a lifetime, you can see how energy-depleting sex can be. Indeed, the Native Americans say, the only way to break the cord is to practice celibacy for seven years!

This may be extreme, but there's no question that sex depends on energy and that energy must be regulated if we're to use it for optimum sex. I used to become annoyed, for example, when one of my former lovers drank espresso before we made love. His nervous system became jittery—his *body* became jittery—and I felt it through his breathing. When I persuaded him to exchange coffee for a vegetable juice cocktail, our sex life improved immeasurably.

I, too, used to think that I could get energy from espresso. It would sure give me a morning jolt, and I'd function as though I were on speed—for a little while. When I came down, of course, I came way down, my energy dissipated and, often, my mood became glum. It's true. I was generating energy, but I was not generating *vital* energy. The coffee was utilizing the energy reserves in my body and spending them. But it's possible to be energetic without using up your reserves; indeed, you'll be replenishing them. Instead of coffee in the morning, try a vegetable juice cocktail. It'll satisfy your craving for coffee and intensify your craving for sex.

———

Your energy is contingent on what you eat.

Ann-Ellen, twenty-eight, is overweight—not fat, exactly, but she could benefit from the loss of ten pounds. What's more, she feels listless, with an appetite for food but not sex, and complains of fatigue. Exercise, which she once loved, now feels like a chore, and rather then go out at night, she'd rather stay home and watch television. It's soon obvious that she's come to see me in hopes of a quick fix.

I ask her about her diet.

"I follow all the rules," she tells me proudly. "A hearty breakfast, no more than a salad and yogurt for lunch, meat, chicken, or fish for dinner, lots of vegetables, no late-night snacks."

"Bread?"

"When I go to a restaurant, I'll have a slice before the meal comes. And of course there's toast with my eggs in the morning."

"Desserts?"

"Plenty of fruit," she says defensively. Then, blushing: "And an éclair for dinner. I can't resist them. But never more than one." She becomes defensive again. "My doctor tells me it's a balanced diet."

In a way, it is. It's not the food intake that's the problem, it's *when she eats what.*

I think of my friend Marcie, one of the most vibrant people I've ever known. She and I have discussed diet many times, and I know that she, too, likes éclairs, meat and chicken, and bread. Indeed, her caloric intake is just as high as Ann-Ellen's. But she eats her "sin foods" at lunch, has roasted oats, fruit, and fruit juice for breakfast, vegetables, rice, and occasionally fish or lean protein at night, but never bread or dessert.

Marcie's eating is in tune with her metabolic clock. She doesn't eat a big breakfast because her metabolism is sluggish in the morning—after all, it's been "asleep" for eight hours and needs time to wake up. She eats her main meal at lunch because, like the sun, her metabolism (just like yours and mine) burns hottest at noon; her body temperature (also like ours) is higher then than at any other time during the day. When nighttime comes, she has given her body ample time for digestion, and her dinner, eaten before seven P.M., will not tax it. She is making sure that her food intake is energy-efficient. She does not gain weight, she bursts with vitality, her sexual pleasure is intense— she is *healthy.*

For Ann-Ellen, I recommend a few adjustments. Two meals a day are all she needs, I tell her, though she can have fruit and fruit juice for breakfast (whoever came up with the notion of three "squares" a day couldn't have had much of a sex life). I advise her to eat her bread, her éclairs, and her protein at lunch so they'll burn off quickest. Digestion, I explain, is a matter of assimilation and elimination. If too much burden is placed on the digestive system—by eating big meals at night, say, or by "grazing" throughout the day, thus not allowing your body to do its housecleaning—the system will not function properly, and at the least your energy level will go down, while at worst you may develop allergies, be immune-resistant, and gain weight.

METABOLIC REGULATION

Anyone who has seen a newborn baby knows that energy is with us from birth. Later, it is up to us to regulate our energy reserves, paying attention to collecting energy, absorbing it, and storing it for times of need. It used to be thought that by the time we are forty, we have "spent" more than half of those reserves, and that by sixty-five our energy reserves are used up. Now we know that such ideas are nonsense, that a woman in her sixties or seventies can be just as vital as a woman in her twenties.

But we must be careful that our energy reserves are replenished, that we eat well, exercise intelligently, and breathe from the diaphragm. The trick is to build from the basics up. If throughout our lifetime we treat our bodies like race cars, jump-starting and screeching to stops, we'll expend energy at a disastrous rate. But if we fine-tune our bodies, recognizing that care means longevity, that maintenance equals vitality, then health—and sexual pleasure—will be ours at any age.

Energy is a primordial force that permeates all living things. It is invisible, yet if we stop to experience it—to "see" it—it is as palpable as wind or fire. We call it the life force. In Sanskrit it is called *prana,* and in Chinese, *chi.* This life force is recognized by all the world's cultures; it moves through and sustains all matter in the universe. It is needed to build and maintain cell structures; to move, to reproduce, to think, to feel. Without it, there is no joy, no sex, no love.

Western medical science says that energy comes from matter—in the case of animals, from food. (Eastern science adds breath to the equation.) As mammals, we obtain energy from the burning of foods—containing carbohydrates, proteins, and fats—combined with oxygen. Some of the fuel is burned immediately to give us instant energy, while some is stored in various parts of the body to be released as energy during times of need—that is, in between meals. Metabolism is all the biological and chemical reactions that are required to carry on life's processes, from the manufacturing of hormones to the building of bones, from breathing to . . . to sex.

———

Each of our some 10 trillion cells requires energy to function. Each cell has within it energy power houses called mitochondria. Within the mitochondria, cellular respiration occurs, the process that produces energy by combining carbon atoms with oxygen in what is known as the citric acid cycle (or the TCA cycle). The citric acid cycle gets its products from the molecules that have been metabolized throughout the organs of the body. Glucose molecules, stemming from the breakdown of carbohydrates (sugar), feed into the TCA cycle. Fatty acid molecules, resulting from the breakdown of fat, also feed into it. Glucose and fatty acids are then transformed into other molecules through oxidation, and the energy released drives virtually all bodily processes.

Some cells have more mitochondria than others. For example, muscle cells contain more of them than fat cells, so lean muscle tissue burns fuel faster and more efficiently than fatty tissue. This explains the need for a low-fat diet, for breathing that will fuel the oxidation process most efficiently, and for exercise.

I've heard people say that they exercise because they want to turn their fat to muscle. Well, fat doesn't turn to muscle—through exercise, it simply disappears.

NUTRITION AND ENERGY MODULATION

You are what you eat—or, rather, what you digest. Digestion is the assimilation of nutrients and the elimination of by-products.

When foods are broken down into molecules that can be used by our cells, the food transforms into energy.

Proper digestion depends on three components: the *timing* of when we eat, the *quantity* of what we eat, and the *quality* of what we eat. To understand why all three are vital, it's important to know something about the digestive process.

Food first enters the mouth, where, I trust in your case, it is carefully and rigorously chewed. (It's amazing how many people simply swallow their food as if they were equipped with a gizzard.) Chewing is an essential factor in good digestion. Not only does it allow you to taste and enjoy, which cuts down on overeating, it also surrounds the food with saliva. Saliva contains a protective substance (IgA) that protects the upper digestive tract from the bacteria found in food, although sometimes the bacteria are so concentrated, or your system so weak, that you get stomachaches or worse despite the protection.

From the mouth, food travels to the stomach by way of the esophagus. Once it has arrived in the stomach, it is further broken down. The stomach produces one to two quarts of digestive juices per day, the main one being hydrochloric acid. In the stomach, protein is digested, minerals are separated from the food, and the bacteria that escaped the saliva are attacked again. The food then proceeds to the small intestine, where most of the digestion and assimilation of nutrients takes place. Here the food mixes with alkaline enzymes in order to increase its absorbability.

The bulk of the matter then proceeds to the large intestine, where it is worked on by microbes (microflora) and the waste products are eliminated. Some microbes promote health; others are toxic and cause disease. Microbes play an essential role in metabolizing nutrients, vitamins, drugs, hormones—and cancer-causing agents. The integrity of the microflora in the intestinal tract determines our health. For that reason, when we overeat, or drink too much, we add to the burden of the microflora and, like a car with inferior oil, we cannot run at peak efficiency.

How many of us have an efficient digestive system? Not many. We have distended stomachs, or complain of heartburn, indigestion, constipation. When we don't absorb the proper nutrients, we get tired, irritable, tense—and as for sex, it becomes unwanted, unappreciated, undesired. Imagine inhaling a box of cookies. Not only will you soon stop tasting them, but your digestive system will be hard pressed to break down the components.

When I first meet clients, the top item on the agenda is to improve their digestion. Once this is accomplished, 90 percent of their symptoms "mysteriously" disappear.

My own sex life improved immeasurably when I went on a special diet featuring a Metabolic Nourisher. I had been eating too much bread and too many starches as a matter of convenience, and my body wasn't digesting them fast enough; I felt bloated all the time. Anatomically, the digestive organs are close to the sexual organs—they're all packed in a small space—so, on reflection, it was easy to see why sex was sometimes painful and uncomfortable. I had too much food in my colon.

Let's come back now to the three components of proper digestion, timing, quality, and quantity. I'll take them one at a time.

Timing

The Chinese system of medicine holds that energy flows through meridians or energy channels in a specific pattern. Every two hours, a different organ dominates. The small intestine, they believe, dominates from one to three P.M. Since it is the organ primarily responsible for digestion and absorption, one to three P.M. is therefore the best time for food to be assimilated. From five to seven A.M., on the other hand, the large intestine dominates. Since it is here that toxic waste is stored, it makes sense that early morning is the most appropriate time to eliminate.

In the Ayurvedic system of medicine—the science of health and longevity—a twenty-four-hour cycle is divided into six segments, not twelve, but the principle is essentially the same. If we follow the energy patterns during the day with respect to our bodily functions, then the body will maintain balance and allow energy to flow freely. For example, because in the mornings between six and ten o'clock we feel most energetic or fresh, what we eat during this time should be cleansing and light so as not to impede that energy. (Test yourself. Many people feel that they need food as soon as they get up, but confine yourself to just a piece of fruit, and see how good food tastes in the next phase of the cycle!) From ten A.M. to two P.M., our metabolic energy is at its highest. Digestive enzymes are up-regulated (activated); food burns most effectively. During this time eat anything you want—but be careful not to eat too much, since you don't want to smother the fire. During the last cycle, from two to six P.M., we feel active and light, in some cases even light-headed. Here we have a tendency to go for sugar and other stimulating foods, since it is the end of the day and we need a boost. Far better to choose food that is stabilizing and moist—"stabilizing" meaning complex foods that regulate blood-sugar levels, and "moist" referring to those foods you do not need water to wash down. Choose fresh fruit over dry fruit, cooked vegetables over raw, baked potatoes over potato chips, lentil soup over lentil salad. Eat soups and protein-rich foods, but avoid stimulating foods containing caffeine or sugar—i.e., coffee and dessert.

The energy cycle repeats itself through the next twelve hours, but instead of repeating the food intake of the day, *don't eat anything at all*. (Water is the exception.) The reason for doing this is that the digestive system needs rest for at least twelve hours daily, and an overnight "fast" is the way to make sure this is accomplished. From a physiological viewpoint, the period from dinner to breakfast is the best time for the body to do its major housecleaning. If you think of the intervals between daytime meals as times for dusting, then nighttime is for sweeping. Not eating before going to sleep allows the metabolic processes to work. If for whatever reason you *must* have something before bedtime, try taking just a glass of water or water with lemon, then herbal teas (without caffeine), and, lastly, milk that has been boiled for three minutes to aid digestion. The nighttime "fast" enables us to digest excess material left from the day, restore cellular function, and repair any damage to the digestive system. Our fat stores begin to break down, too—which is why you would gain more weight by eating at night than you would by eating the same amount during the day.

From the above, it's easy to see that the best time for sex is either early morning or early evening. Our energy and flexibility are highest then; our stomachs are not overloaded; our vitality flows.

Americans, though, are a nation of grazers. We pay little or no attention to our metabolic clock. And since we eat throughout the day, we give little thought to the best time for food—or for sex. It's a pity. Try eating the way I recommend and your health will, I assure you, improve. Have sex at the right time, and your hunger will be for more sex, not more food.

Quality

Our sexual vitality depends on the energy we derive from the food we eat, and the quality of that food determines how much of our vital energy reserves will be restored or depleted. Since 1916, the Department of Agriculture has recommended what food groups are necessary for an adequate diet, and in 1992 officially organized them into a "food guide pyramid," with bread, cereal, rice, and pasta at the bottom; fruits, vegetables, meats, dairy products in the middle; and fats, oils, and sweets at the top. The pyramid is meant as an outline for what to eat each day in what amounts (i.e., more of those at the bottom and less of those at the top).

My vitality diet, however, is somewhat different in that it substitutes beans for most animal-derived protein, limits dairy consumption and substitutes soy products, emphasizes fresh food and whole grains, and eliminates white-flour products. You'll get the same nutritional benefits as you would from following the food pyramid—but overall you'll be healthier and more sexually vital.

The components of food may be classified as micronutrients (vitamins, minerals, nucleic acids) and macronutrients (carbohydrates, proteins, fats), with the micronutrients playing a vital role in the metabolism of the macronutrients. But food is more than just its physical components. It has *essence* as well, just as we do. Fresh food has the life force still present within it, so its nutrients will be easily assimilated, adding to our own life force—our energy.

Let's suppose that the food you eat has been concentrated through dehydration and preserved with chemicals to prolong its shelf life (though not its life force). You will still be eating carbohydrates, proteins, and fats, and if you take vitamin supplements, you will, in Western theory, be "satisfying" your body's basic needs. You'll be getting the right molecules, but as Eastern science has pointed out, and many Western nutritionists agree, it won't be giving you the energy you need. You'll feel heavy and dull—unvital. If you keep eating this way for a long time, you'll feel older than your years, for there will be nothing in your system to restore your energy. That's why I crusade so passionately against canned or frozen foods. I'm against microwaving, too, although here most nutritionists disagree. When you microwave, you're radiating food, but think about it: You wouldn't dream of radiating *yourself* and expect to come out feeling vital. My advice is to stick to fresh foods boiled, broiled, or baked with natural heat. And eat plenty of fresh vegetables. That way, the question doesn't come up at all.

Barbara, a client of mine, was one of those women who didn't believe in conventional ovens. If she cooked, she used a microwave, but she didn't cook much. She had a diet shake for breakfast, diet cuisine for lunch, and a salad for dinner. Well, she was skinny all right, so thin she looked like a prune. Sex is moist, not dry, and Barbara was dry. She did have sex with her lover, but it was always with lubricants.

It's easy to see for yourself the difference fresh food makes. For a week, eat only canned or frozen food. Then eat only fresh food the following week. Take note of your energy, the speed of your responses, your sexual desire. I promise there will be a huge difference. You won't go back to processed foods again. (If this seems too arduous an exercise, prepare some fresh orange juice and then have orange juice from a can, container, or bottle. See how you feel. It's very informative.)

If fresh food is the equivalent of two hundred volts of energy, processed food gives off one hundred volts or less. But simply eating fresh foods isn't enough. Our soil is systematically being demineralized; pollutants fill our air and water. Even when we eat fresh food, we may still not be getting the RDA requirements of basic nutrients, to say nothing of trace minerals like zinc and selinium.

Later I'll be recommending supplements of herbs, spices, and flower extracts to help complete your diet. For now, however, I just want to stress how important good nutrition is. Devitalized food and inadequate amounts of trace minerals and vitamins leave the average person energy impaired. When you're young, you have a natural resiliency that cannot be completely subdued by an improper diet, but as you get older, this is no longer the case, and it becomes obvious how all your functions are linked to your dietary practices.

Correcting your diet, even after years of processed foods and canned juices, can do wonders for your overall health and sexual capacity. If this book does nothing besides convince you to eat better for better sex, it will have achieved a great deal of its purpose.

Quantity

• How many times have you said or heard, "Not right now, darling, I'm too full"?

- How eager are you for late-night sex after a late-night meal?
- How long did it take you to realize that eating *after* sex is pleasurable, while eating before sex is inhibiting?

Obvious questions with obvious answers pointing to one conclusion: Too much food and good sex are antithetical.

When we eat too much, we are directly and grossly interfering with our sexual (and all other) energy. Excess causes loss of vitality, dulls our awareness, blunts our alertness, produces fatigue. Have you ever felt vital after consuming a four-course meal? When I eat that much, I have trouble getting up from the table!

Sometimes we overeat even though on some level we know we would enjoy the food more if we were more moderate. We all know that excess food doesn't translate into additional nutrients, yet sometimes we still eat to excess. The fifth bite of chocolate mousse tastes no different from the first, yet we shovel it into our mouths. Actually, we tend to overeat foods that aren't nourishing, for our digestive systems generally find nonnourishing foods nutritionally unsatisfying and so paradoxically we crave more. By overeating, we put a strain not only on our digestive system, which can't accommodate the plethora of food, but on our nervous system and our *consciousness* as well. Trying to operate on any level—physically, creatively, emotionally, intellectually, or sexually—is far more difficult if the body is trying to figure out what to do with the food it has just taken in.

And yet at the same time, I don't recommend undereating, either, for it leads to a decrease in optimal metabolic capacity. By undereating, I mean not getting enough nutrients for proper metabolic function. This is not the same as cutting down on calories, for caloric restriction can increase life span. (Too much restriction, of course, can decrease it.) I'm talking about skipping meals, and drinking diet soda and coffee in between to curb appetite and take the place of the skipped meals. As you'll see, when we starve our bodies on a regular basis in an attempt to stay thin, we are actually causing stress to our system. Indeed, overdieting by skipping meals is one of the most hazardous threats to women's vitality. What we should strive for, and what this book will teach you to achieve, is balance, a tuning of the digestive system so that you are not consciously aware of the process, but rather feel vital and alive, at full capacity for playing, for thinking, for feeling, for sex.

BREATHING FOR MAXIMUM ENERGY

Until recently, breathing was not particularly associated with health (except that when you stopped doing it, you were dead). Now, thanks to our study of Eastern medicine and Eastern philosophy, we know just how essential to good health proper breathing is.

Even today, though, few Westerners associate breathing with *energy.* To us it is, of course, the mechanical means for moving air in and out of the lungs so that we can replenish our red blood cells with oxygen. Eastern science, however, has added another dimension to the breathing process, *prana*—the life force, our internal flow of energy.

Breathing is the bridge between ourselves and the earth's own rhythm, its own "breath," and human sexual vitality depends largely on the degree to which we are able to absorb the earth's energy into our own through breathing. While this may sound mystical or "New Age" (one of the most inaccurate terms in our language, since much of what we call New Age began with the teachings of Buddha), there is actually a scientific basis for it.

To understand breathing as it relates to energy, we must look at the autonomic nervous system, the purpose of which is to keep our energy in balance. The autonomic nervous system is divided into two branches, the *parasympathetic,* which controls the slowing of the heart rate, the regulation of digestion, and the cleaning of toxins from the body, and the *sympathetic,* which controls our arousal mechanisms and prepares us to take action. The latter comes into play when we are forced into sudden action or experience sudden stress. For example, if we are verbally or physically attacked, the sympathetic nervous system will speed up our heart rate, shoot adrenaline into our bloodstream, cause our palms to sweat, and force us into the instantaneous decision of whether to fight or flee. Both the parasympathetic and the sympathetic systems are affected by the motion of our lungs. When we breathe from the chest, we activate the sympathetic system, but when we breathe from the diaphragm, we balance both systems. Thus the functioning of the autonomic nervous system is directly linked to breathing. When we breathe in, the sympathetic increases ("Take a deep breath," we tell ourselves before entering a stressful situation); when we exhale, the parasympathetic enables us to slow down and increase control.

We breathe in and out anywhere from 23,000 to 26,000 times a day—16 to 18 times per minute. This may be considered normal, but it's not the most healthy. Breathing is a function so automatic that we don't recognize that there are in fact "good" ways and "bad" ways to breathe, and that the way we breathe directly relates to our energy and to our sexual vitality. If we use our diaphragm to breathe, the rate is 9 to 13 times per minute. *This* is healthy.

Breath is the bridge between mind and body. It will go on whether or not you pay attention to it, but if you *do* pay attention (the way you might suddenly pay attention to other "automatic" functions, such as walking or seeing), you can bring it under your conscious control and use it to regulate your vital functions—including your metabolism.

I'll go far more deeply into the physiological aspects of breathing later in the book, but simply to make you aware that there *are* different ways to breathe, try the following simple experiment:

Lie on your back. Relax. Gently place your right or left thumb over your navel and let your hand rest below. Take in a breath as you normally would. As you begin to inhale, your abdomen should expand like a balloon. (Don't *make* it inflate; you're trying to see if it does so naturally.) Exhale. Your abdomen should deflate.

Did it? If so, you are already 75 percent along the path toward revitalizing your metabolism, for you are now breathing from your *diaphragm* rather than your chest, and already you have accomplished a number of beneficial effects:

- You have cut down on the number of breaths per minute, thus enhancing respiratory efficiency.
- You have saved strain on your heart (try taking a number of rapid breaths into your chest and see what it does to your heart rate).
- You have conserved energy.
- You have given a powerful propellant to your blood circulation, sending blood coursing through your system.
- You have greatly enhanced your lung capacity. (For every extra millimeter the diaphragm stretches during inhalation, the lung capacity increases by a volume of 250 to 300 milliliters.)
- You have massaged the glands and organs in the abdominal cavity, in particular the adrenals, located above the kidneys, which are directly responsible for (among other things) the manufacturing of sex hormones.

No one who is not trained breathes diaphragmatically all of the time, but I do and you can, too. It just takes a little practice. This book will teach you the technique for metabolic breathing. It's simple. It's revitalizing. And it enhances sexual pleasure and sexual performance.

EXERCISES FOR SEXUAL REJUVENATION

Margaret, an opera singer, knew how to breathe diaphragmatically; she had been trained to do so because of her singing career. Her diet was good, too, except for an occasional binge just before her menstrual cycle. But she came to me complaining of feeling pudgy and sluggish. Her sex drive, she confided, had decreased; she was often moody and irrationally angry. I saw immediately that she lacked muscle tone except in the area around her rib cage, which she had exercised through breathing. I put her on a full exercise program, and after three weeks she reported firmer thighs, an increased energy level, and better sex with her husband. This was a healthy and successful woman, yet her story emphasized to me how essential a component exercise is to a vital life.

No matter what type of exercise you do, you will improve your blood circulation, bringing nutrition to your cells and glands, rejuvenating the function of tissues, and aiding the proper elimination of waste.

When you don't exercise, you're prey to hypertension, sluggish circulation, and poor cardiac output, leading to shortness of breath and the risk of heart attacks, erosion of muscle tone, and so many other major or minor vulnerabilities that I look at nonexercisers as, literally, at least masochistic and at worst suicidal. (Of course, it's also possible to overexercise, just as it's possible to overdiet. If you find yourself losing your passion for sex—or if you're not looking forward to exercising anymore—cut back on the exercising, but don't cut it out.)

In order to exercise, you need oxygen and glycogen. Breathing, of course, supplies the oxygen; eating supplies the carbohydrates necessary to make glycogen. That's one of the reasons all three components of sexual vitality are inextricably linked.

Exercise is important for the strengthening of muscles (the heart is a muscle, the sphincter is a muscle, the vaginal canal is *filled* with muscles), and muscles contain mitochondria, which as we've noted are responsible for cellular respiration. The mitochondria generate ATP, a high-energy molecule used by all living cells to transfer chemical energy. The more muscle we develop from exercising, the more mitochondria we create to meet our need for energy. We also keep our weight down, improve our posture, balance our hormones, increase our circulation, and help our breathing. Not a bad set of effects from exercise! But beware: Muscles, like every other part of the body, can become overfatigued. We don't want to cause them stress; we want them to be comfortable.

There are exercises for strengthening every muscle in the body, but since this is a book on sexual vitality, the exercises I'll feature all specifically involve muscles essential to good sex. They'll involve organs, too, such as the brain, recognizing the fact that as our most important organ, it is directly involved in sexual pleasure.

Most of us become stiffer as we age. The area surrounded by our hips, which houses the sexual organs, becomes frozen or locked. By exercising the muscles in the pelvic area, tension is released and blood flow increased. As a result, the sexual organs are bathed in nutrient-rich blood and are thus able to be supplied with—and in some cases themselves supply—hormones for sexual functioning.

According to Ayurvedic thinking, metabolic energy manifests itself in the process of digestion in the solar plexus area. If we activate this area, we will increase our metabolic power. In conjunction with the exercises for the lower abdomen (*and* a proper diet and the metabolic breathing technique), these exercises, which activate the solar plexus area, will maximize our sexual vitality.

Vast differences exist between different exercise programs. As you'll see, those I recommend combine both physiological and psychological processes rather than confining themselves just to physical movement. They will not only help you develop a strong physical presence but a body consciousness as well. You'll find that in time you'll let go of certain fears and anxieties, and focus instead on the ease of movement and the freedom of bodily expression the exercises generate.

Before you start any exercise program, ask yourself what your goals are and determine the state of your health. Working with weights, for example, encourages the growth of lean muscle tissue, some of which is lost through diet (another reason diet and exercise work *together*). Aerobic exercise is good for the heart. If you have a health problem, make sure that your program works first to eliminate it. And in all cases, increase the workload gradually. The primary goal is to extend the life span and efficiency of your metabolism—and, by so doing, your sexuality.

When you begin exercising, evaluate your appetite and record your recovery time. If you become ravenous within one to two hours after exercising, cut down on your activity; you don't want to be one of those women who eat so much in compensation for exercising that they actually gain weight. And if after two hours, or even the next day, the idea of another session of exercise seems burdensome, you probably did too much in the first place. The proper amount of exercise produces a high. If you feel depleted and overly sore, cut down but don't cut out.

I'm often asked when the best time is for exercise. It depends on your particular lifestyle. If you're a "morning person," exercise in the morning; if you are most alert at night, do it then. Generally, mornings are best because you don't have the time to think about not doing it (though a slight deterrent is that you may be hungry for the rest of the day and eat too much). Afternoons are worst because work interferes and your blood sugars are low. Exercising in the evening will relax you, but you're likely to be the most tired then (you're also apt to lose the most weight, if that is your goal). It's up to you. The keys are consistency and discipline.

Try any program for at least three weeks, the least amount of time before you'll see a change in your body. If the exercises seem to work, continue for another two weeks before going on to the next level. Make sure you exercise four or five times a week. Less than that and your metabolism won't change. And research has shown that people who exercise four or five times a week lose weight three times faster than those who exercise less.

Again: consistency and discipline. The more you exercise, the easier and more pleasurable it gets. And its effects are wonderful!

————

You'll find a complete three-week starter program for diet, breathing, and exercise at the end of this book that incorporates all of the above. But you may need a bit more convincing before you turn to it.

I want to talk a little about biochemistry. Don't be afraid. It's simple material, and knowledge of it can prolong your life and add radiance to your sexuality.

Chapter 3

THE BIOCHEMISTRY OF HEALTH

Ours is a strange society. We're concerned about health only when it's too late—when we're sick. We have many doctors to treat disease but few to prevent it. We think that we get "worse" as we get older, that frailty is "natural" as we age, that it's "okay" if our sex drive diminishes and our energy wanes as time goes by.

I think of myself as a doctor of health. Women come to see me about health-related issues, from minor complaints like constipation, loss of energy, lethargy, mild depression, and so on to chronic conditions such as stress-related lower-back pain, PMS, migraines, and yeast infections. All come with a lack of sexual vitality because those other conditions permeate their days and they can't even *consider* sex. However, all of these women go away with renewed sexual interest. Their feminine essence is enhanced. So I'm convinced that the prescription in this book is vital for your health. It is to be taken *before* you get sick, and if followed, it will keep you healthy far longer than you thought possible.

The essence of good health lies in biochemistry, the science of the composition, structure, properties, and reactions of matter as it affects our biological processes. The sum of these biological processes is what creates our metabolism. Our diet, movement, breathing patterns, and mental state all contribute to this. Therefore, we have a good deal of control over our health through our habits.

The key to our biochemical processes is the liver, our metabolic hotel. Its functions include detoxification, storage, and metabolism.

As a detoxifier, the liver processes food, drugs, toxins, and chemicals—anything that comes through our digestive system—and can either neutralize or convert them to be excreted in nontoxic form. For example, the liver's detoxification pathway changes a toxin that is initially fat soluble to one that is water soluble for easier excretion by the kidneys.

The liver also stores vitamins and minerals (B12, A, D, E, K; iron, zinc, manganese, copper, and molybdenum), combines niacin and glutamic acid to make it possible for us to tolerate glucose, and combines other nutrients to make antioxidants that protect our other organs.

As a metabolizer, it manufactures cholesterol, the basic molecule from which our adrenal hormones and our sex hormones—estrogen and testosterone—are produced. It is also responsible for the metabolic control of carbohydrates and proteins, and it regulates levels of glucose and amino acids in the blood.

The liver is responsible for the breakdown of sugar between meals and during times when food is not available, such as when we're asleep. It absorbs oxygen and nutrients from the blood to keep metabolic reactions working properly. It is the most important organ in the body when it comes to health. If it functions improperly, so do we.

Yet many of us abuse it. We overload it with fats or alcohol, bombard it with chemically processed foods, saturate it with sugar.

Eating "clean" food, rich in minerals and vitamins, is the way to a healthy liver. To do this, I advise adding special nutrients, including bioflavonoids, vitamins C, E, B1, B2, B3, and B5, and folic acid, to aid the liver in detoxification. Herbs, too, support liver functions, which is why my diet includes bitter herbs, beet greens, milk thistle, dandelion, and ginger. Occasionally, I recommend herbs containing iodine to aid in thyroid function.

And avoid eating late at night or grazing throughout the day. The "hotel" needs periodic housecleaning or it will fall into disrepair.

Maintenance not only of the liver but of complete biochemical balance is something you can do every day; it should be as natural as walking.

———

Biochemistry was the subject of my doctoral dissertation at Case Western Reserve, and the root of my studies was liver metabolism. I got to look at all my bad dietary habits of the past—caffeine, occasional drugs, excessive sugar and fats—and for the first time realized what my poor liver had had to endure. No one ever told me how to clean and regulate my liver; no one ever told me how important my liver was to my sexual vitality. I was in such bad shape that I developed sun spots, sometimes referred to as *age* spots—and this while still in my twenties! (These spots were a clear indication of sluggish liver metabolism.) My menstrual cycle was all screwed up; I had all sorts of vaginal problems. Sex? Forget it.

In the course of my studies, though, aware of the metabolic significance of sexual vitality, I put together a plan. For a month, I took dandelion and milk thistle to clean and regenerate my liver. I drank fresh juices daily, often several glasses. I ate beans, rice, herbs, and enough vegetables to become a walking garden. Since I love sweets, I didn't cut out cookies but ate the fat-free varieties from natural sources. I made sure my foods were without chemicals or preservatives. I started to exercise. I learned to breathe properly.

And in the first two months of detoxing, my sex drive disappeared! In fact, I felt no vitality whatsoever. I was plagued with fatigue and intense sugar cravings.

But an exciting thing was happening to my body. My eyes became clear. My skin glowed. My vaginal problems disappeared. My menstrual cycle became regular. My puffiness went away. Even my sun spots vanished, although this took six months.

Eventually, I dared to add protein to my diet—fish, chicken, or eggs. And one day—with a joyful vengeance—my sex drive reappeared, and it was like having *new* sex, sex I had not experienced before.

I got my Ph.D. I got a life.

————

What are the foods that give us energy—and why?

Carbohydrates come from grains, fruits, vegetables, and legumes—these are what I call "favorable carbohydrates." (They also come from refined sugar, cakes, pastries, and white-flour products—what I call the "unfavorable carbohydrates.") We get food energy ultimately from the sun. Plants take water and carbon dioxide from the air and capture the energy from the sun, forming carbohydrates and releasing oxygen. Carbohydrates are our quickest source of energy and assist the body in metabolizing proteins and fats—fats, for example, require carbohydrates for their breakdown in the liver.

Fats come from a number of sources; they can even be produced from eating an excess of carbohydrates. We need fat in our diet primarily for membrane function and lubrication, but a superabundance is unhealthy, sometimes disastrously so.

Foods rich in fat are milk and butter, cheese, vegetable oils, and meat. Our heart uses fatty acids as fuel, but they don't burn easily, tend to clog our arteries, and overload our cells, which then lose their vital energy. Far better to eat tuna, salmon, wild game, avocados, almonds, pecans, pumpkin, and pine and sunflower seeds as sources of fat. But, alas, the "bad" fats make up 30 to 40 percent of the American diet. Why do we like them so much? Because they taste good and satisfy our appetite. That's why fast foods are so much in demand. But beware! Fast foods are dangerous.

Next to water, *proteins* are the most abundant substance in our bodies. They are our major building blocks, essential for the growth and development of all body tissue. During digestion, protein is broken down into amino acids by stomach acids mixed with enzymes from the pancreas. The amino acids are then absorbed by the intestine and travel in the bloodstream to the liver, where they are used to synthesize new body proteins to be used for the formation of hormones, enzymes (substances necessary for many biochemical reactions), and other substances used to regulate metabolism. In times of starvation, protein stored in the body can be broken down and used for energy. When excess protein is consumed but not utilized, it is converted to fat in the liver.

The major sources of protein are meat, fish, poultry, eggs, milk, soy, and legumes. Again, make sure you don't eat too much of them. Unlike other energy fuels, they have no storage forms independent of function, and too much protein in the system puts a strain on all affected organs. They are, in effect, a fuel of "last resort."

Our conventional notion of a balanced diet is to combine all the major food groups at every meal—at breakfast, for instance, we're taught to eat fruit, eggs, and toast. But this approach does not take into account the fact that everyone's digestive system works differently, and that canned vegetables and fruits are radically different from fresh. Studies have shown, for example, that hormone levels of insulin were different after subjects consumed a meal of fresh beans versus canned beans.

My recommended diet includes whole grains, vegetables—crucifers, roots, and leafy greens—fruits, nuts and seeds, sea salt (not table salt, which is stripped of potassium), seafood, sea vegetables, beans, and free-range eggs. You can add some more hormone-free dairy and a little meat, but eliminate processed foods entirely. More than six thousand synthetic chemicals are officially condoned for use in the food industry, some with known carcinogenic effects. The human system recognizes chemicals as toxic agents, and ingestion of these agents causes the system stress. The liver then can't do its work properly, leading to increased aging and deterioration of the immune system, to say nothing of the depletion of the sexual organs.

What about sugar? Again, moderation is essential. White sugar, the kind to avoid, is devoid of the vitamins and minerals necessary for it to be digested. So we rely on our nutrient stores for the digestive work, and thus our stores become depleted. Complex sugars, on the other hand—those found in whole grains, vegetables, and fruits—have the requisite vitamins, minerals, fiber, and water for proper digestion. Another reason to avoid white sugar is because it suppresses the immune system by making the pancreas secrete abnormally high quantities of insulin and causes the adrenal gland to become depleted because the body reacts to sugar overload the same way it reacts to stress. Since processed carbohydrates like white flour, candy, pastries, and cookies are "unnatural," the body treats them as it would toxins. Eat too much sugar and you're prone to many of the ailments associated with decreased vitality: decreased libido, candidiasis, diabetes, heart disease, obesity, and atherosclerosis.

The body needs to borrow essential vitamins and minerals to metabolize sugar, so it robs itself of its essential reserves. This can also lead to food cravings and eating binges, since the body needs to replenish what it has lost to sugar. The excess is converted into fat, called triglycerides, by our liver, and the result is often depressed moods and nearly always decreased sexual desire. I've noticed that my own libido disappears with the last cookie. I'm satisfied with sugar, but it's much more fun to be satisfied sexually.

———

I've said that herbs are an essential supplement to your diet. I recommend flower essences, too.

Flower essences are liquid formulations made by combining flowers with water, the idea being that the flower will transfer its "energy" to the solution. One theory is that flowers contain a subtle, vibrational energy that resonates with human feelings and emotions. Another is that the essences have the ability to alter electrical impulses that affect messenger molecules in the body's psychoneuroimmune system. While some of this may sound "New Agey," I believe there is a scientific basis for the effectiveness of flower essences, and that both mind and body are eased by their use. Each flower has its own unique properties, making it suitable for treating specific emotional or psychological problems, such as fear, anger, anxiety, and even low self-esteem.

Flower essences are key parts of traditional healing systems in India, Tibet, China, Japan, and Indonesia. The Vedas, among the oldest written texts, talk of treating illnesses with flowers, and the Aborigines of Australia still use fresh flowers in hot-coal saunas, a practice some ten thousand years old. Flower essences do not cause chemical changes, but nevertheless affect the nervous system, and thus emotions, thoughts, and feelings.

The appendix contains a list of flower essences and their specific benefits, including properties that deal with immune system disturbances. They are not a mandatory part of my program, but I encourage you to try them.

———

We have seen that the biochemical body depends on good nutrition and that good nutrition is most effective when combined with proper breathing and exercise. It's time now to become more specific and to discuss biochemistry as it pertains to disease prevention, stress reduction, radiant aging, and sexual pleasure.

THE BIOCHEMISTRY OF DISEASE PREVENTION

Many diseases stem from the wrong use of sexual energy, for it is the primary energy of mind and body. Most psychological disorders are based on the inability to form healthy relationships and are thus largely sexual in origin. It stands to reason, then, that the right use of sexual energy is the key to health.

Everything we do directly affects our sexual vitality. Our bodies are a network of interconnecting organs that are affected by our environment both externally (air, water, and land) and internally (the food we ingest, our enzymes and our hormones). To be healthy, all of our systems, not to mention the interaction between mind and body, must be in balance and must flow smoothly. If the balance is askew or the flow is interrupted, disease results.

Our immune system is the first line of defense against virus, bacteria, cancer cell formation, and other invaders—in a word, disease. It includes the lymphatic vessels and organs (thymus, spleen, tonsils, lymph nodes), white blood cells (the primary defenders), and other specialized cells and serum factors. Since many diseases come from pathogens in our environment, the immune system's job is to battle these poisons and, essentially, eat them up.

When our immune system is compromised—by poor diet, by lack of exercise, by fatigue, by alcohol or drugs—it becomes weakened and we are correspondingly more vulnerable to the pathogens that create disease. How do you know if you have a healthy immune system? Ask yourself how often you catch a cold or how often you feel run-down or tired. If the answer is "a lot," change your diet, your exercise program, your way of life—or all three.

Here are the warning signs:

Stage one: Slight changes in your body like fatigue, weakness, lethargy, overly emotional responses to ordinary events.

Stage two: Colds, flu, swollen lymph nodes.
Stage three: Increase in blood pressure, blood sugar, and choles-
terol and triglyceride levels.
Stage four: Disease.

My advice: Watch at stage one, pay close attention at stage
two, feel the urgency for change at stage three, avoid stage four.
There are two essential steps to take in battling disease:

1. Strengthen the immune system through diet and exercise.
2. Upgrade the body's ability to remove toxins by strengthening the liver.

The diet that will help you do this is the one you'll find in
this book. Add herbs and vitamins—specific ones; their healing
properties are listed in the appendix. And exercise, not only following the ones I've included here, which are primarily for sexual vitality, but in many different ways (walking and biking,
swimming and jogging are among them), for exercises increase
the immune function by bringing new oxygen into the cells.
Too much exercise, on the other hand, can exhaust the body of
nutrients, so stop when you feel tired. I'm appalled to see
women huffing away on a StairMaster, faces red and sweaty, for
I know how much they'll have to eat to compensate and how
needlessly exhausted they'll feel for the rest of the day.

As for upgrading the liver, cut down on sugars, fats, and particularly large amounts of alcohol. Eat right, breathe right,
exercise right, and the liver will soon be cleansed and operating
at full efficiency.

THE BIOCHEMISTRY OF
STRESS REDUCTION

According to Dr. Phil Neurenberger in *The Quest for Personal
Power: Transforming Stress into Strength,* stress is "a state of auto-

nomic imbalance, characterized by unrelieved or excessive dominance of either arousal or inhibition, or a complex unbalanced interaction of the two."

In other words, stress occurs when we are out of balance. This imbalance leads to biochemical imbalances within our organ systems.

When we experience stress, our bodies' reactions come from either sympathetic nervous system dominance (characterized by arousal) producing a fight or flight response, or from a dominant parasympathetic nervous system (characterized by inhibition) producing a possum response. Sometimes there is a mixture of both. In the case of sympathetic dominance we may get sweaty palms or heart palpitations, become irritable or angry or forgetful; we may experience sleeplessness, back pain, neck stiffness, digestive trouble. On the other hand, if the parasympathetic system is dominant, we may become withdrawn, unable to face the situation, close down or become depressed, which themselves lead to sickness and disease. Ultimately, we can control these reactions; they come from the autonomic nervous system, which controls the functioning of the internal mechanics of our bodies that don't require conscious input. When we digest food, when our heart beats, when our kidneys secrete urine or our liver regulates metabolism, it's all controlled by the autonomic nervous system, so obviously any disruption of that system caused by stress can lead to malfunctions of the body's ordinary processes.

Under stress, the body is in a constant state of imbalance, and its functions, like fighting off environmental toxins or digesting and metabolizing food, can be temporarily shut off.

Biochemically, when we undergo stress, the activation of the sympathetic nervous system causes the adrenal glands (located above the kidney) to secrete stress hormones: catecholamines and corticosteroids. These hormones cause the body to release its stored energy, thereby elevating fat and cholesterol levels in the blood. They break down the cells of the intestinal tract, depress the immune system by inhibiting the function of white blood cells, decrease lymphocyte production, and can cause shrinkage of the thymus gland. Remember: The adrenals are responsible for manufacturing sex hormones, and when the body is under stress, their production stops. Of all the sexual inhibitors, stress is the most powerful. Biochemically, when the parasympathetic system is dominant, we find functional loss due to underutilization of the body's resources. Muscles begin to atrophy due to loss of use. For example, the heart may become enlarged due to lack of exercise. Illnesses associated with a dominant parasympathetic nervous system may include chronic fatigue, depression, and possibly some forms of cancer.

If you're feeling stressed (and there may not always be an immediate, recognizable cause; the stress may be "free floating"), my program will help. Proper diet creates emotional and physical changes leading to biochemical balance. Fruits and vegetables contain phytonutrients that balance hormone production. Foods rich in calcium, like beans, nuts, and all manner of greens, are particularly good aids to relaxation (add lemon to the vegetables; it will draw the calcium out). Seaweed nourishes the nervous, immune, and hormonal systems. Gotu kola stimulates the brain tissues, thereby expanding consciousness and comprehension and calming the mind. The best of all known herbs for restoring the body under stress is ginseng.

Exercise, of course, allows you to work off some of the inner tension caused by stress, since it affects both body and mind. It is also useful in balancing the nervous system, not only to relieve tension caused by sympathetic dominance but also to activate our system when we are stressed because of an extreme parasympathetic dominance.

And breath is particularly important. Deep, diaphragmatic breathing puts the body in a state of relaxation and will provide your cells with the extra oxygen needed for rebuilding themselves.

Stress is a relatively new phenomenon brought on by the rhythms of a society geared toward speed, production, and success. Fifty years ago it was a word applied to bridges, not to people, and maybe if we got rid of fax machines, television sets, cellular phones, E-mail, and call waiting we could ease our own lives enough so that a special program would be unnecessary. But that is fantasy. Stress is due to how we view modern life and we must address it.

THE BIOCHEMISTRY
OF RADIANT AGING

The body degenerates when its ability to repair itself falls behind the breakdown of its own biochemical processes. We've all known young people who seem old and old people who seem young; in fact, chronology is not as important in the aging process as maintenance of the bodily functions.

To most people, progressive degeneration of bodily functions seems to be the norm with aging. The process accelerates if we lead a toxic lifestyle and live in a polluted environment. As we age, it seems that repairs take longer—but why? Scientists have speculated that either the body is generating more *free radicals* or the body loses the ability to dispose of them.

Free radicals are unstable oxygen molecules with unpaired electrons that, when paired with other molecules, alter their chemistry. They are generated during the metabolic process and have the capacity to attack membranes, the enzyme systems, even your DNA. They can also develop in the body from exposure to toxic chemicals in the air, food, or water; radiation from X rays and sunlight; cured meats, alcohol, herbicides, drugs, nicotine, and stress. Free radicals are highly toxic and are normally sequestered by substances called antioxidants as soon as they are produced. (Research has shown that they may contribute to cancer and heart disease.) Most are eliminated by our system, but some are not. Overproduction of radicals results in a cascade effect and more free radicals are formed.

Antioxidants—defined as any substance that delays or inhibits oxidative damage to the tissues—come in the form of a variety of enzymes, particularly superoxide dismutase, catalases, and glutathione peroxidases. They exist as part of the liver's detoxification system. Other antioxidants, like coenzyme Q10 and melatonin, are also manufactured by the body and serve as natural antioxidants. Our antioxidant defense system needs vitamins and minerals taken from our diet, particularly selenium, copper, zinc, vitamin E, and vitamin C.

Oxidation is what happens when something rusts. My program will prevent the rust. No matter how far along you are in the aging process, *start now!* And remember these tips:

- Overnight fasting enhances the immune system by allowing the regeneration of intestinal cells, which fight off foreign invaders. So don't graze.
- Eat less, live longer. By decreasing your caloric intake, you will lengthen your life span.
- Raw fruit juices and vegetable juices are the best source of organic vitamins and minerals.
- Limit fats to 20 grams or less a day. Polyunsaturated fats produce free radicals. When you do eat fat, choose cold, pressed, unrefined oils like olive, peanut, or sesame.
- Avoid processed foods as well as other foods that have chemicals in them—sweeteners, artificial coloring, etc. Our environment is toxic enough as it is. Why add to the burden placed on your liver?
- Include bulk raw fruits and vegetables in your diet. They contain the best source of organic substances that repair and nourish cells.
- Include fiber by eating whole grains and legumes. They keep the bowels clean and act like a broom to sweep out toxic substances.
- To the vitamins mentioned above, add carotenoids, particularly beta-carotene. Other carotenoids are found in green leafy vegetables.
- Flavonoids, found in fruits and vegetables, neutralize free radicals and potentiate vitamin C.

- Milk thistle, green tea, ginseng, gotu kola, and ginkgo biloba, among others, are herbs that have been shown to retard the aging process.
- Flower essences that help as well are pretty face, self-heal, hibiscus, peppermint, snapdragon, and alpine lily.
- As noted, deep diaphragmatic breathing increases oxygen capacity and metabolic efficiency while cleaning away toxins. Relaxation breathing reduces stress.
- Exercise to increase muscle mass (weight training) and to decrease fat (aerobics). The bromide "Use it or lose it" is true for all parts of your body—and particularly for the sexual organs. It has been proved, for example, that vaginal atrophy is more prominent in women who do not have sex.

THE BIOCHEMISTRY OF SEXUAL PLEASURE

It's amazing how much has been written about men's sexual performance (how to get it up and keep it up) and how little about women's. Aphrodisiacs are prescribed to give men more stamina in bed; ginseng ads are pitched at men, and it is men who are advised to eat oysters. But this book is intended for women, and there's no question that certain foods, vitamins, and minerals will enhance *women's* sexual pleasure—yours and mine.

My own feeling is that aphrodisiacs should be taken (I can't resist) with a grain of salt. Oysters may indeed be an aphrodisiac, but only if a person is zinc deficient. Calming foods—warm milk, honey, sweets made of ghee, sweet fruits—will ease stress and so increase sexual appetite. Caviar and red wine can stimulate sexual response, but probably because you ingest them at special occasions, often with someone you love. What's simply food in one culture is an aphrodisiac in another (I can't imagine being turned on by bird's nest soup, but the Chinese swear by it); truffles, I'm told, work for pigs, but while they're delicious, I haven't felt an increase in desire after I've eaten them—and they're expensive!

My point is that a satisfactory sex life requires more than overhyped supplements; it requires a healthy body, which depends on nutrition, exercise, and breathing technique. If your body is balanced and not nutrient deficient, your sexual energy will be at its peak. In order for you to be sexually active, there are specific organs and glands that need to be nourished, and my program is specifically geared to nourishing them.

We'll discuss hormones in depth in the next chapter, but let's look now at how hormones relate to sexual function.

The pituitary gland is located at the base of the brain, just below the hypothalamus, and makes a hypopituitary consortium that is the most complex and dominant portion of the entire endocrine system. It is responsible for regulating the functions of other glands throughout the body, including (for our purposes) the adrenal glands, which govern our level of fatigue; the thyroid, which directly affects the libido; and the ovaries. Any deficiency in the pituitary causes underdeveloped sex organs, early menopause, and impotence (in men) and frigidity (in women).

The adrenal glands produce a small but significant amount of sex hormone and, for proper functioning, need vitamin A, the B vitamins, vitamin B1, pantothenic acid, niacin, vitamins C and E, the mineral magnesium, and unsaturated fatty acids like those in flaxseed oil. Without them, the adrenals will become exhausted, resulting in a lack of sexual vitality and a decrease in function. You'll get enough of all of them, however, if you follow my program.

The thyroid gland is correlated with sexual desire and sexual strength. The B vitamins and vitamin E, and the minerals iodine, zinc, and copper, are essential for the production of its hormone, thyroxine.

The ovaries secrete two hormones, estrogen and progesterone. Insufficient estrogen causes, among other conditions, delayed sexual maturation and a lack of development or shrink-age of the breasts and genitals. An imbalance of progesterone causes irregular bleeding, water imbalances, and erratic changes in mood and behavior. The B vitamins, vitamin E, folic acid, niacin, and zinc are essential for the proper functioning of these hormones.

The sex hormones are made from cholesterol, which is pro-duced by the body, and in most cases we don't have to take in more of it. At the same time, though, we do not need to omit all cholesterol-rich foods from the diet, as long as they can be easily metabolized. Nutrients that help the metabolism of cho-lesterol are the B complex vitamins, vitamins C and E, magne-sium, manganese, zinc, and lecithin.

Just as good nutrition is essential for sexual radiance, so a bad diet will harm it. Drugs? They might increase sexual pleasure for a while, but they'll soon destroy it. Alcohol, cigarettes, caffeine, carbonated drinks, processed foods, and highly refined sugar are all sexual depressants. Some antidepressants, antihypertensives, and tranquilizers will also decrease sexual desire and pleasure; so will birth-control pills, which have been shown to interfere with the metabolism of carbohydrates and fats and to destroy certain nutrients, including several B vitamins, folic acid, and vitamins C and E. They are also shown to affect thyroid function. If you're on the Pill, my program will be especially beneficial.

The appendix will tell you what herbs, flower essences, vita-mins, minerals, and foods will help you maintain peak sexual vitality. For the moment, though, remember these general pieces of advice:

- Avoid white-flour products. I've found that women have dessert in place of sex. Biochemically, the release of sera-tonin from eating carbohydrates satisfies the pleasure center, so it's chocolate cake or sex. Your choice.
- Seaweeds help with thyroid function and are rich in miner-als like iodine, calcium, and zinc. Drink miso soup. Eat sea-weed salad.

- Avoid adrenal-depleting foods like coffee, chocolate, and foods containing refined sugar.
- If you can, avoid unnecessary use of oral contraceptives, as they deplete thyroid function as well as sexual energy.
- If you have low thyroid function, limit your intake of broccoli, cauliflower, and cabbage.
- Eat fresh fruit, leafy vegetables, whole grains—indeed, the entire vitality diet.

The basis of sexual pleasure is hormones. You know how vital estrogen is to women and testosterone is for men; in the next chapter you'll learn how hormones work and why the vitality program will keep them flowing.

Chapter 4

THE HORMONE MESSENGERS

Hormones are the most important energy-support system we have. Everything in the body functions or malfunctions based on our hormone production, secretion, and circulation. And regular sex is one of the best ways I know to keep hormones flowing freely. But sex isn't essential. Ultimately, the mind has more effect on hormonal flow—far better no stress than no sex.

In my own case, when I first got to Cleveland, I was terrifically stressed and had had no sex for four to five months—my entire body shut down. I stopped menstruating. I gained weight. My metabolism slowed down. I was continually depressed.

At my doctor's suggestion, I took the synthetic hormone Provera—a chemical form of progesterone—to bring on my periods. But the drug made me more depressed, and I put on more weight and got yeast infections, hardly the solution I was looking for. Good God! I was supposed to be a nutritional biochemist, and I was about to go to the Olympic center to begin my research with the Taekwondo athletes.

It was only when I met a man at the Olympic center (I still don't know why he was attracted to me) that things changed.

We arranged to meet in New York six months later, and I went on a program of exercise in the evenings—the best time if you want to lose maximum weight. I took baths with juniper and cypress to get rid of the cellulite. I used oil of sandlewood on my neck to revive feelings of femininity. I cut out all forbidden foods. My periods didn't return immediately, but they came back before my lover arrived (he was amazed at "how radiant" I looked), and I've been having regular periods and regular sex ever since. You may think that I overdid it, but remember that I was young and sex-starved—and he *was* attractive.

I don't want to claim that sex alone will regulate menstruation and hormones, but for sure it's a great balancer. During sex, many substances are exchanged by way of mouth and penis to mouth and vagina, as well as through the pores of the skin. Hormonal balance is multifaceted, and intercourse can be a stimulus for all systems to integrate. Think how each system is intertwined. When the vagina and penis engorge with blood and engage with each other, they activate centers throughout the body, stimulating hormonal production and circulation. The brain is also stimulated by sex, especially the pituitary gland, located at its base, the master gland that signals many other systems to operate. And our breathing affects our limbic system, which in turn affects our pituitary.

———

Marilyn, age fifty, comes to see me, anxious and depressed. She is in what doctors call perimenopause, that state just before actual menopause sets in, and the time between her periods is getting shorter, twenty-four days instead of her usual twenty-nine. Her moods are as erratic as her periods; she is frequently angry—indeed, she seems miffed when I tell her that she is experiencing a hormonal change.

"I know that!" she barks. "What it really means is I'm getting old."

"Just because your hormonal balance is changing doesn't mean your life has to change," I assure her. "Getting enough exercise?"

"I work out three or four times a week. Forty minutes on the treadmill and StairMaster. Light weights on alternate days."

"Perfect!" I say. "Diet?"

"I eat fat-free foods."

"Meaning?"

"Fat-free cookies, low-cal pasta, diet soft drinks—you know. Nothing harmful. But it's driving me crazy. I have this enormous craving for sweets."

Anything beneficial? I wonder, but I say nothing aloud. "How's your sex life?"

"What sex life? I'm fat as a house despite the fat-frees, so my husband won't look at me. Besides, I have as much desire for sex as for a root canal. Anyway, it's normal not to want sex at fifty, isn't it?"

She is only slightly overweight. Sexual radiance, I remind myself, has a lot to do with attitude. She doesn't *feel* radiant, although she is in fact extremely attractive.

"I'm not sure what 'normal' means," I say. "But I know plenty of fifty-year-olds who love sex. Let's take a look at your diet. It's probably there that the problem lies."

Her diet, as I suspected, is deficient in foods that help regulate hormones. I explain that she's eating too many carbohydrates (the fat-free foods contribute), which get converted to fat by way of the hormone insulin. It's putting stress on her body.

"You need to add vegetable protein," I tell her. "Soy and legumes."

She brightens. "I like Chinese stir-fry."

"Try some animal protein, too. At lunch. Maybe three ounces." This will help with insulin responses and weight gain. "And eat some tofu, drink some soy milk."

At home she adds soy milk to her cereal and for lunch makes what I call a phytoestrogen delight—vegetables, spices, and tofu. On my advice, she eliminates her daily quota of six cans of Diet Coke, which has been depleting her body of vitamins and minerals, especially calcium. I introduce her to Kukicha tea, a Japanese twig tea she buys at her health-food store, and, after consulting with her doctor, put her on the herb Vitex, meant to nourish the pituitary and help restore menstrual regularity.

It usually takes a few months for such a program to work, but in Marilyn's case the results are quickly apparent. Because she came to me at the onset of perimenopause, and because she religiously adheres to her regimen, progress is rapid. She begins to lose weight almost immediately. Her menstrual cycle regulates itself at twenty-eight days. Her sex drive returns. Her black moods lift.

Her last visit is six months after her first. She is radiant. "Now, *that's* normal aging," I tell her.

————

We have a group of organs and glands that make up the endocrine system. These organs and glands—the adrenals, the thyroid, the pineal, the ovaries, and so on—produce, synthesize, and secrete hormones, the chemical messengers that tell the body how to behave. Many scientists believe hormones to be the most important chemicals in the body. Without them, we literally could not function.

The word *hormone* comes from the Greek *horman,* meaning to urge on, and in a sense that's what hormones do: "urge on" the nervous system, the immune system, and the reproductive system, among others, so that they perform healthily and appropriately. Hormones are the master regulators. The endocrine glands send messages to the brain, which in turn "alerts" the hormones to enter the bloodstream, and depending on which particular body function they are intended to affect, they then "stop off" at their designated cells, much like a super-sophisticated Federal Express system, delivering the correct hormone to the correct location.

While men maintain a high degree of hormonal consistency throughout their lives, women's hormonal levels go through two phases each month: (1) when hormones from the pituitary gland stimulate the follicles in the ovaries to grow in size and number and excrete estrogen so the stimulated follicles give rise to an ovum, and (2) when the ovum is released into the fallopian tube and when, if no fertilization takes place, menstruation occurs.

Far greater hormonal changes occur during menopause. Interestingly, this seems to be more of a problem among women from Western cultures than from others. We Americans seem to look on menopause as something to be dreaded—that "change of life" that takes us closer to death, a change that takes anywhere from one to five years. But in the Black Hills, Native Americans celebrate the change for three days and three nights! My friend Ike Sayther West told me that the women simply go to sacred caves in the Hills, where they use nature's products—crystals, herbs, and mosses—to aid the process. Menopause is thus celebrated with a ceremony honoring the transition from one phase of life to another.

Ike married into the Eagle Clan, well respected for what they know about healing. The eagle itself symbolizes balance; if it loses a feather from one wing, it will lose a feather from the other. "In your society you think of healing in terms of taking something out," she told me, "removing something from the body, a germ or a cancer. To Native Americans, though, this is very imbalanced. If you take something out, you must put something back. If you have an endocrine imbalance, say, from ovarian insufficiency, a grandmother would ask: 'What have you given away? Your femininity? Your femaleness?' If the woman gets her femaleness back, there is no void to fill with disease."

Part of the aim of this book is to "put something back"—herbs and essences that restore femininity, vitality sapped by nutritional imbalances, sexual feeling eroded by anxiety and stress. If you give away sex, either indiscriminately to men or to

a too-pressured society, you give away one of your greatest gifts.
It must be replenished.

———

Anything that causes an imbalance in either the total amount or
the ratio of the secreted hormones can cause a wide range of
health problems. For menstruating women, the most common
of these include premenstrual tension, excessive menstrual
bleeding, and menstrual irregularity. In general, on a physical
level, most hormonal problems in women are the result of low
or high estrogen and progesterone, an imbalance between the
two, or low or high levels of pituitary hormones.

Our menstrual cycle has its own rhythm, corresponding to
the earth's energy fields and the moon's dominance over the
tides. Women's cycles are also influenced by the type of relationships we enter into. College roommates or female cowork-
ers often cycle at the same time each month. Women who have
sex regularly stimulate endocrine blood flow and hormonal
secretion (it's also a good way to maintain a well-lubricated
vagina). During the cycle, we become intuitive as to what we
want or need. During ovulation, for example, some women
express a greater desire for sexual intercourse. But we don't
need to make love to someone else for this balance. We can love
ourselves.

You can see that artificially altering the cycle (by using birth-
control pills, for instance) will interfere with these instincts, but
there are times when hormone therapy is needed—when a particular organ is secreting too much of a hormone, too little, or
none at all. Overall, though, I think hormone therapy is used
too often, especially around menopause. Far better to depend
on diet, adding vitamins, minerals, and herbs. Indeed, in many
cases, I've seen women with many symptoms of hormonal
imbalance recover with a change in diet alone.

———

Since this is a book about sexual vitality, any in-depth discussion of the endocrine system is beyond its scope, but some endocrine glands directly (or even indirectly) affect our sexual activity and should be at least mentioned:

1. Hormones from the *pituitary gland* influence, among other things, rate of growth, rate of metabolism, ovulation, and lactation. Deficiency in the pituitary can cause underdeveloped sex organs or early menopause in women, and often a drop in the level of sexual desire. The pituitary secretes a hormone called ACTH (adrenocorticotropic hormone), which plays a part in the adrenals' production of androgen, a hormone some consider to be even more important to sexual vitality than estrogen.

2. Hormones from the *pineal gland* influence moods, sleep/wake cycles, and appetite. The hormone melatonin, in particular, affects sexual desire in that the more you secrete, the less intense your sex drive. Since melatonin is released from the pineal gland in inverse relationship to the amount of light you're exposed to, patently—for sexual desire at least—you should soak up the sun.

3. Hormones from the *thyroid gland* influence virtually all our body's systems, which is why people with an underactive thyroid are often fatigued, depressed, and lacking not only in sexual vitality but even in the desire for sex. The thyroid produces the hormone thyroxine, which, when biochemically converted to triiodothyronine (T3), is responsible for stimulating nearly every cell in your body.

4. Hormones from the *adrenal glands,* as I mentioned before, synthesize other hormones, including sex hormones, and, if functioning well, act as a buffer against stress, surely the most powerful of all sexual depressants, barring actual disease. Perhaps the two most important hormones secreted by the adrenals are cortisol, which is activated in response to stress, anxiety, and hypoglycemia, and DHEA (dehydroepiandrosterone), an adrenal androgen, which is the precursor of the sex hormones testos-

terone and estrogen. High levels of DHEA are found in vibrant young women, but they're greatly affected by smoking and stress, since under stress our bodies don't manufacture as much DHEA, having to concentrate instead on producing what is often an excess of cortisol. As we age, we're told, the level of DHEA decreases—thus the current rage for DHEA tablets. My own view is that if we keep stress low through diet, exercise, and breathing, we'll reduce strain on the adrenals, leaving them free to manufacture their own DHEA without a need for supplements.

5. Hormones from the *pancreas* regulate our blood-sugar concentrations. The pancreas secretes the hormones insulin and glucagon into the bloodstream, the latter when we need glucose taken out of storage, such as in between meals, and the former after we eat and need to store glucose in our cells. Both hormones help regulate our ups and downs during the day. When they're not regulated (as, say, when we pig out on pastries), we have a surge in insulin and a drop in glucagon—with a corresponding drop in sexual desire.

6. Hormones from the *ovaries,* estrogen and progesterone, regulate our fertility and our physical sexual characteristics. Insufficient amounts of estrogen, for example, can delay sexual maturation or cause shrinkage of the breasts and genitals, though this may not coincide with a lack of libido. It's true that at menopause production of estrogen and progesterone decrease, and that the amount fluctuates during our menstrual cycles, but the female body has the capacity to make adjustments in hormonal balance throughout its lifetime. For instance, it's important to note that other body sites manufacture estrogen and progesterone, which is why my sexual vitality diet is concerned with the adrenals, digestive system, kidneys, and liver, even though they only indirectly affect sexual performance.

Here's a brief listing of the endocrine gland hormones and the nutrients they require:

Endocrine Gland Hormones and Nutrient Needs

GLAND	HORMONES	NUTRIENT NEEDS
Pituitary	Growth Luetenizing Follicle-stimulating	B-complex vitamins, Pantothenic acid (B5), niacin, vitamin E, zinc
Adrenal glands	epinephrine/ norepinephrine DHEA, cortisol	Vitamin A, B-complex vitamins, Pantothenic acid (B5), thiamin (B1), niacin, vitamins C and E
Thyroid	thyroxine	Iodine, B-complex vitamins, thiamine (B1), vitamin E, copper, zinc, vitamin A
Ovaries	estrogens, progesterones	B vitamins, folic acid, vitamin E, zinc and nia- cin, essential fatty acids

As you can see, when we speak of hormones and sexual function, we are not only speaking of sex hormones, but other hormones as well that indirectly have an effect on sexual vitality. If one organ or gland doesn't function efficiently, it can create problems for the rest of the system, and since our sexual organs are not used for actual survival, they are the first to be compromised when any part of the body becomes dysfunctional.

Can they be revived? Of course. One key is diet.

———

All plants contain chemicals—collectively referred to as phytonutrients or phytochemicals, "phyto" meaning plant—that have an impact on our hormones. These chemicals are manufactured by plants throughout their life span but especially during the early stages of growth. Each plant category—cruciferous vegetables, for example, including broccoli, cabbage, and cauliflower—has its own particular chemicals, which affect our systems in different ways. This is why we need to have a varied diet.

Certain phytonutrients work as hormonal balancers, since they are used in the hormonal systems of the plants themselves. Plant-source sex hormones are being used now as an alternative to synthetic hormones and have been proved safer in many cases. How these plant chemicals are used in our bodies depends on our hormonal messengers, and also on the functioning of the enzymes and receptor sites in the endocrine glands.

Let's see how all foods, plants among them, work on hormonal function.

Foods and Hormonal Function

FOOD	FUNCTION
Simple sugars	Decrease libido. Deplete adrenal hormones.
Fiber (whole foods)	Influences estrogen metabolism. Increases sexual stamina.
Fats	Decrease libido and sexual performance. Increase circulation of potentially harmful hormones.
Seafood	Essential minerals that increases libido (i.e., zinc). Some contain essential fatty acids that provide moisture to skin, vagina, and bladder, and are particularly important when estrogen levels decrease.
Legumes (mung, lentils, chickpeas)	Source of estrogenlike compounds.
Fruits	Source of bioflavonoids, which regulate hormone production.
Vegetables	Contain many antioxidants, and phytonutrients that manufacture sex hormones. Some contain essential fatty acids for hormone production.

Seaweeds	Richest source of minerals for endocrine glands—especially thyroid, which controls libido; also contain estrogenlike compounds.
Soy products	Contain compounds that can balance the body's need to manufacture its own estrogen.
Grains (oats, barley, brown rice, wheat)	Regulate blood-sugar levels, increasing stamina. Contain estrogenlike compounds that balance hormones.

And here are some of the chemical compounds found in different kinds of plants.

Plant Compounds Found in Foods That Balance Hormones

CHEMICAL COMPOUND	FOOD
Isoflavones	Soybeans, alfalfa, fennel, parsley, licorice, chickpeas, mung beans, whole grains
Lignans	Linseed, rye, buckwheat, millet, sesame seeds, sunflower seeds, soybeans, whole legumes, whole grains like oats and barley, vegetables and fruits
Isothiocyanates and Indoles	Cruciferous vegetables: cabbage, broccoli, turnips, watercress, radishes
Allylic compounds	Garlic and onions
Carotenoids	Orange-yellow vegetables
Coumestans	Soy, alfalfa, mung beans, red beans, split peas, olives
Flavonoids	Vegetables and citrus fruits

Finally, here are some of the herbs that support hormonal balance.

Herbs That Support Hormonal Balance

HERB	FUNCTION
Vitex	Balances the ratio of the hormones estrogen and progesterone by acting on regulatory hormones in the pituitary gland.
Don quai	Contains high phytoestrogens. Regulates menses and relieve hot flashes, vaginal dryness, and fatigue.
Black cohosh	Helps maintain vaginal integrity. Estrogen promoter.
Wild yam	Corticosteroid manufacturing agent (used to make synthetic progestin—dioscorea villosa). Used for premenstrual tension.
Ginseng	Decreases the production of stress hormones; therefore, keeps sex organs vital. Increases libido.
Gotu kola	Most important rejuvenative herb in Ayurvedic medicine. Stimulates the synthesis of collagen, the first step in tissue repair (uterus repair after menstruation). Strengthens the adrenals and purifies the blood.
Licorice	Stress buffer herb. Works on adrenals. Take with caution. Licorice stimulates progesterone production while decreasing estrogen. Contains isoflavones.
Ginkgo biloba	Increases brain circulation, which may affect pituitary and pineal glands in regulating sex hormones.
Dandelion root	Detoxifying herb, for breast, mammary, and lymph glands, liver and gallbladder. Good for detoxification from meat diet and excesses of fatty and fried foods.
Ginger	Metabolic stimulant. Aids circulation of hormones and assimilation of vitamins and minerals necessary for endocrine function.

My program takes account of all of these, but clearly, with study, you can mix your own combinations.

———

Remember the autonomic nervous system, with its sympathetic and parasympathetic branches? Each branch stimulates the organs, and when you breathe and exercise, hormones are released from those organs, helping the bodily functions to continue to operate.

In my program, we use breathing and exercise as a means for taking conscious control over our autonomic nervous system. If we regulate our breathing and the amount of our exercise, we can regulate our bodies and minds via both the sympathetic and parasympathetic branches. Certain endocrine glands receive a rich supply of neurons from both branches, and the activity from these neurons regulate hormonal secretion. For example, epinephrine and norepinephrine are manufactured by the adrenals during stress; insulin and glucagon, as we've seen, are manufactured in the pancreas, and so on. When we regulate our breathing patterns and exercise correctly, we can change many of the physiological responses.

When we're stressed or scared, we breathe from the chest, and by inhaling and exhaling rapidly, we cause the adrenals to produce adrenaline, a fine response if you're about to be attacked by a lion, but not something you want to do on a regular basis.

Diaphragmatic breathing, on the other hand, gives a powerful propellent to blood circulation, thus boosting the circulation of hormones, sending them coursing through the system without causing extra work for the heart. Too, diaphragmatic breathing massages the adrenals—indeed, all of the female reproductive organs—and by so doing increases the flow of hormones into the ovaries, where their major work is done.

———

So far, I've talked mainly about chemistry and biology. But there's patently more to sexual radiance than that—there's the spiritual side. Much of this aspect of sexual pleasure was first discussed by philosophers in the East, and there is a lot to learn from them. Even if we have no wish to incorporate their entire philosophical regimen into our lives, we can find pleasure in their mythology and learn many things from their physical and spiritual view that can deepen the way we understand our sexuality.

Part II

—

DECODING LESSONS FROM THE EAST

$\mathcal{T}$HE ENERGY SYSTEMS

According to the philosophies of Yoga science, within ourselves we have seven energy centers, called *chakras*—"wheels"—that govern our physical, emotional, mental, and spiritual well-being; thus, they provide the foundation for sexual vitality.

From a neurophysiological perspective, the chakras represent nerve plexes from the spinal column and endrocine glands that connect with internal organs. The first chakra is located in the area of the coccyx, the base of the spine, and is called the coccygeal plexus. It encompasses the perineum, rectum, and prostate gland. The second, below the navel, is related to the lumbar plexus, the female reproductive organs, and the male testicles. The third is associated with the solar plexus, adrenals, and pancreas, and is the seat of our metabolic center. The fourth is the "heart chakra," which is connected to the cardiac plexus, thymus gland, and pericardium. The fifth relates to the thyroid gland located at the level of the throat, connected to the vagus nerve and cervical ganglion. The sixth is associated with the pituitary gland, and the seventh the pineal gland.

Since this is a book on female sexual radiance, I'll be concentrating on how to activate the second and third chakras, though you should be aware that vitality in one area generally means vitality in all.

By now, it will not surprise you to know that the second and third chakras are affected by diet, exercise (the leg lifts in my program are particularly effective), and breathing, but this chapter will concentrate specifically on how and why my program works on balancing the chakras, and how and why your sexual responses will become tuned with their energy so that the flow of female essence will increase your capacity for sexual union, bringing to it creativity and spirituality.

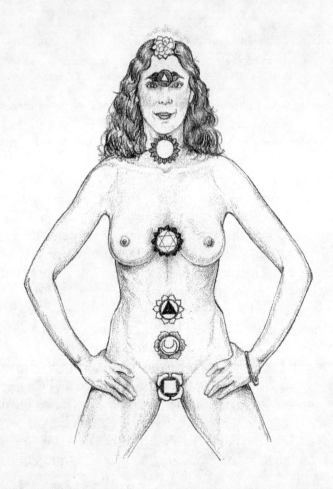

While the chakras correspond to physical plexes throughout the body, according to the philosophy of yoga science and Taoism, they are also centers of energy—the "life force" or "prana"—that, in essence, *are* our vitality.

Kundalini—energy—resides in the first chakra (the one at the base of the spine) and waits to be awakened. The life force generated when it awakens is contained in the cerebrospinal fluid, which travels upward through the inside of the spinal column, passing through the remaining chakras and through thousands of energy pathways called *nadis* (or "meridians" in the Chinese acupuncture tradition).

Tantra, a meditative tradition of self-mastery that brought art, ritual, and all scientific, mathematical, astrological, and alchemic knowledge into the realm of the spiritual, teaches that one way kundalini can be released is by the practice of *asanas*—yogic positions that include movement and breathing—whereby sexual impulses become the pathway to cosmic consciousness. I'll expand on Tantric sex in the next chapter; here it is enough to say that asanas teach us to hold our sexual energy rather than release it, to explore our senses rather than subdue them. Breathing and meditation are essential. The clutter and chatter within us and without become muted. The partners concentrate solely on the fulfillment of their mutual pleasure. But the pleasure is not only physical; it is also a means of spiritual awakening. Tantric sexual union blurs the delineation between man and woman. It is a state of bliss in which the sacred and profane, the corporal and spiritual, the finite and infinite are merged into the ecstasy of being one with the cosmos.

In the process, the woman is all-important. She is, in effect, the link between the actual and the transcendent; she is both flesh and blood and ethereal, woman and Woman. She enjoys freedom and detachment and is regarded as the embodiment of *Shakti,* the active female principle in kundalini. (The man is the embodiment of *Shiva,* the active male element.) When kundalini sleeps, we are aware only of our earthly situation.

When she awakes, we are carried into the source of light (in modern terms, into those vast dormant parts of our brain capable of bringing us into higher consciousness). True ecstacy can only be obtained mutually, between man and woman, yet paradoxically the woman must be active, independent, self-motivated. Ultimately, hers is the power to create—she is the bearer of life, capable of the creation of others and of self-creation—and it is no wonder that she is considered sacred.

Remember, kundalini does not pass upward through the chakras in a straight line. At each stage it encounters different energies that block its progress, and it must take on these energies so that positive and negative forces, existing in us all, can be merged.

The word *kundalini* is now fashionable in the West, but few people really understand it. Like all Tantric concepts, it is not easily mastered. In one of my classes, a woman came to me and said she had kundalini sex. I asked her what she meant. She told me that during intercourse she saw brightly colored stars and her body began to shake. This is, I'm afraid, the antithesis of kundalini. The colors of the stars are not the colors of kundalini, which are not known in the Western spectrum. And if she was shaking, it means she was tense, whereas when kundalini rises, the body is totally relaxed, the breath regulated. The woman simply had a splendid orgasm.

———

The first three chakras are the basis for our animal instincts—matter of survival, sex, and self-maintenance—but the next three, beginning with the heart chakra, are less tied to the physical world than to the spiritual realm, the realm of more evolved consciousness. Actually, the heart chakra is represented by a six-pointed star, symbolizing the interlocking of two triangles, the one pointing down representing the female energy, the one pointing up the male.

The seventh chakra is the point at which we attain the wedding of the spiritual and the sensual, and thus full self-awareness and realization. We are on the threshold of enlightenment.

Ultimately we want to work through the lower three chakras and not get stuck in them so that we can enjoy the pleasures of the world and still be free to achieve a full spiritual life.

In the first five chakras, the five elements of earth, water, fire, air, and ether (different from the Chinese elements, which replace earth and ether with wood and metal) blend with the senses of taste, touch, sight, sound, and smell, and all are connected to the internal organs through the autonomic nervous system and the nadis. It sounds easy to say that we must allow the energy to rise through the chakras, much as hot air rises to the top, but to actually do it is difficult. Many potential physical and psychological roadblocks exist at each level, and it is possible to get stuck in any one of them. If, for example, we are stuck at the third chakra, which among other things represents the fire element, we are likely to have psychological issues of aggression, incompetence, overachieving, and anger. Physically, we may have digestive problems, hypoglycemia, sluggish liver function, and insomnia.

In other words, chakra energy manifests itself on the level of both the body and the mind—and on the spiritual level as well, which we will get to later in the chapter.

We don't, of course, operate in one chakra at a time. Issues at the various levels are dealt with simultaneously, not sequentially. One may predominate, but all function continuously on some level.

We've noted that energy travels from the first chakra, located at the base of the spine, to the highest. Think of our energy system as going up a staircase and stopping at each floor. On each floor we find different offices with different "business" concepts. Energy can move freely up the staircase, but it can also get trapped in one of the offices and thus not fully or effectively reach the offices on the higher floors. As noted, kundalini may not travel without impediment.

Let's say our energy stops in the second chakra, the lumbar plexus, known as our pleasure center. Energy must flow freely in it if we are to be sexually vital, but if the energy cannot flow upward, we are prone to many sex-related ailments, both psychological (promiscuity, sex addiction, unmodulated sexual energy, gluttony, overreliance on alcohol) and physical (lower-back pain, vaginitis, urinary tract infections, cystitis, and so on).

Proper diet, exercise, and breathing will ensure that this chakra, like all others, functions properly, siphoning off the requisite amount of energy for its use, but allowing the rest to travel upward to the higher chakras.

———

I spoke earlier of prana, the life force that is the essence of all living things. Breathing is the vehicle that carries prana along, since the process of manufacturing energy can continue only as long as we continue breathing. Breath is very key to life. If it stops, our bodies die. It connects us with the consciousness of both mind and body. It brings energy to our cells through our nerves, veins, and arteries (our nadis), those branches that keep our metabolic functions up and running.

The breathing process itself is a neuromotor action; inhalation and exhalation are performed with the help of the nervous system. When we are in the womb, the pranic force flows into us via the lungs of the mother through the umbilical cord, which is at the navel center. When we enter the world, our own lungs take over, but the navel center remains key to our prana, for it is still the center of our digestion and is the origin of the pranic channels, the nadis. The navel center energizes and empowers all other systems of the body; its chakra is associated with fire, both metaphorically and physically, since it is the seat of metabolism. Patently, the navel center is vital in maintaining sexual vitality, which is why my program is specifically designed to stimulate energy at this center in order to create a pranic force.

I will get into the specifics of my metabolic breathing technique later. For now, it's enough to know that rhythmic breathing makes all the molecules in the body move in harmony. It is used to purify the autonomic nervous system and to give vitality to the centers of the body—the chakras. Learn to regulate your breath, and you will maintain energy. Indeed, you will be able to "feel" the energy as it enters the chakras—and if you can feel it, you can control it. Great sex is not possible without controlled breathing. It conditions both the physical and the spiritual. It is the stuff of life.

We saw earlier that our digestive capacity determines the assimilation of nutrients and the elimination of toxins. Western nutritionists look at the physical components of food—fats, proteins, carbohydrates—and try to compose a properly balanced diet among them. Eastern nutritionists (and philosophers) add the component of prana and concentrate on those foods that give us the most energy. My diet does this, too, for if it is true that the navel center and its attendant chakra is associated with fire, and fire is the element that transforms matter into energy, then foods that fuel this fire are essential to metabolism.

———

All the healing forces available to us originate in our metabolic balance. Those of us who have not gained access to these forces will be subject to the "normal" process of aging, to say nothing of an increased proclivity for a variety of diseases. You may master all sorts of diet fads and fancy exercises, but unless they regulate your metabolism, all the work will be in vain.

You can test your own metabolism in terms of the fire element, which governs the third chakra. If it is balanced, you will feel energetic, assertive but not overly aggressive. You will feel confident and passionate; your moods will be stable, your sex drive moderate. However, if you are out of balance, you will feel anxious, lethargic, either overly passive or overly aggressive. You will be quick to anger, quick to cry. Indigestion will be frequent and your sex drive will either be nonexistent or quick to surface and be depleted. By balancing the third chakra, you will regulate the first two as well, since it is higher up the ladder and can eliminate blockages in the lower two.

Are you overweight? If so, there's probably a malfunction in your metabolism, which may not be changing food into energy. If you carry excess padding in your abdomen or if your posture is affected by disproportionate fat, you may not be properly activating the third chakra and will have to change your diet.

If you lose energy quickly when you exercise, have shortness of breath, get easily depleted and run down, or crave stimulants such as coffee or sweets, you should probably change your diet in order to adjust your metabolism.

Fire is the fuel for life that ignites will to action. Fire in our body keeps us warm, active, energized, able to put into action our thoughts, our desires, our longed-for pleasure and joy. When we're cold, our energy is blocked instead of radiant. When our metabolism—our fire—is strong, we glow with vitality, with life.

———

As we grow older, our physical and psychological states change and, as a result, so do our needs. As our physical state changes, so does the way we eat, but at any time of life, our eating is related most of all to the first three chakras. We ingest food from the earth, the first chakra element, then transform it into energy in the second and third chakras. Eating nonpolluted and fresh food—"live" food—is the first step toward establishing a healthy environment for our first three chakras, and though for many of us it is impossible to eat farm-fresh food every day, at least we should be conscious of what we do eat and try as much as possible to avoid the processed foods, canned foods, and refined sugars that sap the vitality from the nutrients, and, in turn, from ourselves.

Various types of food have various vibrational levels in that they have different energies themselves and produce different types of energy when eaten. As they are processed chemically by the body, different foods support the different organ systems associated with each chakra. My basic diet will pretty much ensure that each organ system functions optimally, but it is fascinating to note how closely individual foods and their psychological and physiological effects are tied to the individual chakras.

The table on page 84 shows how it works.

From this list, you can readily see what foods will specifically aid your sexual vitality. But all chakras must be tended to nutritionally, since, as we shall see in the next chapter, sex is by no means solely a physical function, but encompasses all five senses, as well as the brain, the mind, and—indeed—the soul.

———

Just as there are specific foods for the individual chakras, so there are specific exercises.

Exercises for the first chakra involve the feet, the backs of the legs, the hamstrings, and the knees. (Here, as with the other chakras, specific exercises will be demonstrated later in the book.)

For the second, exercise the pelvis, the legs from knee to hip, and the lower back.

For the third, exercise the abdomen and the area from the anus to the heart.

For the fourth, exercise the chest area mostly through standing exercises involving the arms and upper body.

For the fifth, exercise the neck and throat.

For the sixth and seventh, exercises should not be so much physical as mental. Yes, you can do headstands, which will bring blood to the brain, but meditation, thought (or the absence of thought), contemplation, and the slow development of these chakras to the point of spiritual attunement enhances not only sex but all aspects of life.

Working with the body really teaches you about the chakras. Wherever there is blockage—an emotion held in, a too-

CHAKRA	1	2	3	4	5	6	7
Physical function	elimination of solid waste, stability, groundedness	elimination of liquid waste, fluidity	digestion, assimilation, acid/alkaline balance, burning fuel	nurture, breathing, circulate oxygen, immunity, receiving	swallowing, expression, eliminating poisons, receiving	rectifies faults in other centers	kundalini energy merges
Psychological function	fearlessness	sexuality	willpower	love/ compassion	ingenuity	imagination	perception
Associated symptoms	colitis, tight hamstrings, paranoia	cystitis, low-back pain, vaginitis, jealousy	digestive problems, sugar metabolism disorders, anger, inferiority	circulatory disorders, cancer, immune disorders, selfish, overly emotional	sore throat, eating disorders, stubbornness, pessimistic	headache, overthinking	none, ignorance
Foods for optimum function	legumes, root vegetables, nuts and seeds	all fresh juices, liquids	complex carbohydrates	green leafy vegetables	fruits	herbs, working with the mind	fasting

powerful inhibition, a sickness—the corresponding body part will be locked. When I was young, a friend tried to teach me the Marinera and the Festejo, two Peruvian dances of seduction. I couldn't get them. My hips wouldn't let go; my pelvis seemed made of stone. Since I was a good athlete, there seemed no reason for my inability to master the relatively simple movements, yet I was a robot. "You're holding something in," my friend told me. "Don't think. Just *move.*"

I let myself go, just danced to the music without thought and without wondering how I looked. In moments, the movements came naturally. But it was not until some time later that I recognized that the movements—gyrating hips, thrusting pelvis—were sexual, and that my inability to dance was simply a manifestation of a sexual inhibition inculcated during childhood. I mastered the dance in a day. Sex took a little longer.

Chapter 6

*T*HE ART OF TANTRIC SEX

Tantra is the science of inner life, a four-thousand-year-old discipline leading to physical, mental, and spiritual self-mastery. Literally, it means "a web," an intertwining of all aspects of the human condition—physical, psychological, spiritual, emotional—in which sexual fulfillment is to be found. My aim is to bring Eastern sexual discipline to the West, but it is beyond the scope of this book to explain all the facets of Tantra. Patently, there is much more to Tantra than sex, but one of its overall goals is to take sexual energy and transform it into spiritual energy, which ultimately leads to liberation. Phil Nuernberger, an experienced Tantric mystic, puts it this way: "Tantra is discipline, but the Western mind rebels at discipline. The Western mind wants pleasure, pleasure, pleasure. The purpose of Tantra is spiritual union, not physical or emotional pleasure. Sexuality can be a powerful tool, just as diet can be a powerful tool. But for the Tantric mystic, sexuality is an instrument, not a path. The path is inner discipline." (Perhaps a more accurate way to describe the principles here is to speak of "Tantric union," for Tantra itself involves rituals and an underlying philosophy that go far beyond the realm of this book.)

Still, Tantric yoga is the only form of yoga that teaches the value and importance of sensual experience in the transformation of actions into inner awareness and ultimately selflessness or enlightenment. All other yoga schools, seeking the same goal, insist on the monastic life—renunciation, detachment, and asceticism—but Tantra is not this way. Its aim is to fully discover and realize the Known, and thus it deals with understanding the sciences and experiencing the pleasures of life. Sexual pleasure is to be used to assist the woman in her yogic practices, spiritual cultivation, and search for divine ecstasy. As we saw in the last chapter, if Tantric union is to be achieved, the body must be cleansed (through breathing) and the mind cleared (through meditation). Everything must flow. Woman and man must merge into One. And even if you do not believe in the Oneness of the universe and do not understand the cosmic resonances of Eastern philosophy (few people do; true understanding takes a lifetime of study), there is much here that can be applied to sexual radiance in our own Western bodies and minds.

Perhaps the element I like best is the fact that in Tantric union, the woman is to be honored and adored. It is she who is the mother-womb and is therefore endowed with all aspects of life: creative, benign, sublime, sensual, horrific. As we've seen, the kundalini Shakti—coiled-up energy—resides within all of us. When kundalini Shakti is dormant, we are aware only of earthly things and earthly functions, such as orgasmic sex. However, when we are able to arouse her, she travels through the chakras and we are able to move to another plane, where mystic as well as physical union can take place.

While in some Eastern philosophies sex is considered an impediment to enlightenment and women who indulge in sex are maligned as promiscuous or "unfortunate" (there are many analogies here to the West, where some people still consider it "sinful" for women to enjoy sex), in Tantra the woman is celebrated, even worshiped. And the culmination of that worship is an offering of sexual pleasure that guides the woman to the spiritual realm and transforms sexual passion into divine energy.

Liberation comes from within; there is no dependence. Both man and woman have a mutual journey to blend strengths. Since we have a desire for sex, use that desire to lead you toward enlightenment. Tantra preaches mutuality.

———

There's no question that sex and energy are interrelated—indeed, sex *is* energy, both physical and mental. I know a fifty-year-old couple who make love every day, which does *not* mean that the man ejaculates each time (this is a basic Tantric teaching: Ejaculation expends energy, while conservation of the semen replenishes it throughout the body), but that they have learned to breathe together, and that they have learned to use sex not as a means to the goal of orgasm, but as a means toward meditation and oneness. In other words, their sex is not goal-directed ("Can he hold back until I come so we can come together?") but rather aims at the calm transfer of energy between the couple, an entrainment that will spread to all other bodily organs, leading to health and renewed vitality.

They don't lie back after sex, they tell me, "spent" and "satisfied." Rather, they feel a surge of energy that carries them throughout the day, since they usually make love in the morning. The energy of sexual intercourse has flown upward throughout their chakras, affecting their immune systems, their hearts, their souls.

In Tantric theory, sex can either enhance or deplete energy. Ejaculation depletes male energy through the expenditure of semen, whereas menstruation depletes female energy through the loss of another vital fluid—blood. Women advanced in Tantric practices can actually reduce or stop menstrual flow. Western doctors would think they were bizarre, but essentially the idea is the same as in nonejaculation: to conserve energy and send it throughout the body.

———

My teacher, who was a Tantric master, used to say, "You are the architect of your life and you decide your destiny." He was talking about self-mastery, control over the physical, emotional, and spiritual aspects of our lives.

Self-mastery requires self-knowledge, self-discipline, and systematic training, none of which can be achieved without diet, proper breathing, and meditation. It sounds simple, but our habits, built through our lifetimes, often get in the way. I studied with several Eastern masters and was struck by the fact that they did not seem to have aged in a "normal" fashion. They were far more energetic than Westerners their age; their skin looked younger; they had better posture and walked with more assurance. All of them followed strict regimens of diet, meditation, and breathing. I have simply adopted some aspects of their programs to Western—and specifically Western women's—needs.

Self-knowledge, discipline, and systematic training—let's look at them one at a time.

SELF-KNOWLEDGE

A simple definition of self-knowledge is the ability to recognize what is useful to you and what is not, combined with the ability to understand *why* you act as you do and *react* as you do. By becoming aware of your own habits and recognizing the way your mind works, you can begin to approach your unconscious, and what you might have described as your "crazy" behavior now takes on meaning and sanity.

Louise, for example, came to me complaining that every time she and her husband began to make love, she had to urinate. The several doctors she consulted could find no medical cause; I tried to find the psychological one.

One of the best tools in developing self-awareness is breathing. I'll bet you don't know which of your nostrils is dominant when you breathe, and I ask you—now—to become aware of it. Ah, the left. Now consciously transfer to the right, even using a finger to block the left if necessary. What's happened is that you've become aware of something that you do unconsciously thousands of times during the day; your mind is suddenly focused on breathing to the exclusion of everything else.

I asked Louise to perform the same simple experiment, and told her that self-awareness was the essential first step toward self-knowledge. "Now," I told her, "when you begin to make love with your husband, become aware of what you feel. It's like breathing. Something is going on unconsciously that you must bring to the surface."

Soon she reported back. The feelings that lovemaking aroused were not sexual, but rather those of anger.

"You're pissed off at him?"

"Damn right!"

"And you wonder why you have to go to the bathroom?"

She looked at me and smiled. "Ah."

On her next visit, she announced success. "I was able to tell him why I was angry at him. He understood, and we talked it out. Our lovemaking was the best it's been in years."

"And urinating?"

Another heart-lifting smile. "It never entered my mind."

I know that awareness of the physical aspects of our lives can lead us to an awareness of our mental processes.

One good method for developing self-knowledge through self-awareness is to keep a journal, not necessarily for every activity, but for those you think are significant. Kathy, one of my clients, had consistent migraines. I recommended that she write down her food intake and correlate it with the headaches—what had she eaten just before they occurred? Soon the answer was clear. Dairy foods! Before her headaches she would have cream in her coffee and cheese on her pasta. When she cut them out, the headaches disappeared.

Not everybody has this reaction to dairy food, but other foods can cause problems as well. Awareness of diet can lead to knowledge of behavior. After you eat sugar, do you get depressed? Do you feel angry after two glasses of wine? Do you get sleepy after meals? If you can interpret your physiological state, you can often interpret your psychological one, and if you learn to become aware of your actions, your thoughts, and your habits, you will be able to change useless or self-destructive behavior, whether it be physical or mental, and concentrate on what is good for your body—and your soul.

SELF-DISCIPLINE

"Discipline" sounds punative, a type of punishment. But when taken in conjunction with willpower, it becomes the second factor in self-mastery, a positive—indeed, an essential—element in a fuller, more realized, more vital life. No long-lasting life change is possible without discipline. No long-term job can be accomplished unless you apply it.

Sometimes, of course, discipline *does* seem like punishment. "I've cut out all sweets entirely," a client who adores ice cream told me recently.

"Good for you," I said, eyeing her dubiously. "Do you feel better for it?"

"Better?" she cried. "It's *torture!*"

Precisely. Discipline does not mean a kind of Prussian adherence to a regimen that will "do you good." It does mean the application of willpower to point you toward a desired goal. Willpower means mind-strength. Discipline, its sister, means the ability to apply that strength when needed. When it comes to dieting, for instance, start simply, cutting down without cutting out. When it comes to exercise, work up a sweat, not a lather. If the price of discipline is pain, you're overdoing.

And remember, discipline is mental as well as physical. A positive mind-set is a prerequisite. The word *can't* creates an obstacle in the mind that reinforces failure. "I *want* to do it. I *can* do it. I *will* do it" will take you a long way toward achievement. It takes discipline to think positively. But the rewards are multiple.

SYSTEMATIC TRAINING

An adjunct of discipline, systematic training simply means that you need to set aside time to exercise and meditate *and to do both within your capacity.* It means dieting for a lifetime, not simply for a week or two, *but with the flexibility to deviate from time to time depending on external influences.* You must make a commitment to yourself consistent with your lifestyle and follow a program that has qualities you enjoy and that do you no harm physically or psychologically.

In my program, I ask women to chart their present schedules to find out the optimum times for eating and exercise. Often this means breaking decades-old habits (eating lunch on the run, exercising only on weekends) and building new ones. My program starts slowly, then goes on to increments of thirty minutes for eating and ten minutes for breathing and exercise. The building of new habits is the goal of systematic training, for the main difference between me and you is our habits—and habit can be the greatest obstacle to self-mastery or the greatest tool to achieve it.

———

If you accept the premise of modern psychology that our behaviors are conditioned by seeking pleasure and avoiding pain, you can see that habits are created from patterned behavior, behavior that becomes systematic and over which you no longer need to have conscious control. We come to regard our habits as a normal part of us, and we don't ever consider the possibility of changing them.

Take diet. When I ask my overweight clients what they eat, their answers are varied but the message is the same:

"I don't eat much."
"I try to stay away from sweets."
"I don't eat much meat."
"I stay away from fats."
"I'm into fruits and vegetables."

These people are not consciously lying, yet their records belie their statements. They don't realize how much "much" is, how far they "stay away" from sweets (or eat fatty foods in compensation), what else they're "into" along with fruits and vegetables. When I point out to them what they're *really* eating, and how ingrained a habit it's become, they're astonished and vow to change. What they must do, of course, is to become self-aware. People get used to their habits and don't see them anymore. Self-mastery restores their vision.

Some habits dull our awareness, blunt our alertness. *Seeing* these habits and correcting them effect wonderful changes in our state of mind, metabolism, and health. When we're sick, we tend to regress psychologically and function on a primitive, self-protective level—a habit not unique to us but common to everyone on earth. When we're regressed, we can't interrelate. When we can't interrelate, we're incapable of satisfactory sexual union.

When we're very old or dangerously ill, our primitive habits are probably protective and valuable. But if we mistreat ourselves when we're young, if we don't work to build different, healthful habits, then we'll never discover the full glory of sex or the excitement and contentment of a relationship built on openness and mutual pleasure.

———

There are five steps to creating useful habits:

1. *Recognize* that you need to change.
   If you begin a self-investigatory journal, you'll more easily be able to see what habits have inhibited you in the past.

2. *Identify* the habit you want to create.

In your journal, write down your goal and the means to the goal. If the goal is sexual vitality, one habit you might adopt is the overnight fast. Stick to it for twenty-eight days. After that, you'll find it's become a habit, and you won't want to go back to large dinners and/or bedtime snacks.

3. *Be systematic.*

Make sure you practice the new habit at the same time each day. If you want to add metabolic breathing to your life, pick an optimum time of day to do it, and stick to it for at least twenty-one days. If you find it causes problems, remember Step 5!

4. *Be consistent and persistent.*

It takes twenty-one to twenty-eight days to create a habit, so for the first month or so you'll have to act consciously and maintain your schedule. I worked with a woman named Phyllis who had eaten two pieces of toast, with butter and honey, every morning for thirty-five years. To switch to a glass of fruit juice as a substitute took enormous discipline. Now she tells me that the thought of anything heavier than juice for breakfast turns her stomach.

5. *Be flexible.*

The ability to change *within* a habit, when appropriate, will paradoxically make any action more easily habit-forming. Thus if the time of day, the kind of juice, the strenuousness of the exercise becomes a burden, then be flexible. If you become too rigid with rules and regulations, tension builds. If you overtighten a guitar string, it will break; if you tighten yourself too much, your good intentions will break. You must have the *will* to change habits or develop new ones, and in most cases you won't feel the need to be flexible, but you should enjoy yourself! Useful habits should bring joy not only in their effects but in performing the habits themselves.

Does all this apply to sexual vitality? Absolutely. Self-mastery is essential to sexual vitality, as are its components.

How many times do we pay attention to our physical or mental preparation before we have sex? Not many, I'd guess, at least after the wooing process is over. When we're "sure" of our partner and know that sex is there for the asking, we either "just do it" or we don't, depending on our mood. Many married women, women with long-term lovers, or women with constant multiple partners complain to me that often they're "simply not interested" in sex, or wish their husbands/lovers would stop bothering them.

These women are looking at sex as a physical act resulting in a pleasurable spasm, which may or may not be worth the effort required to achieve it. What they are *not* doing is regarding sex as an exchange of energy with their partners, an experience that cultivates vitality not only in the sex organs but in the wholeness of both selves—mind, body, spirit. As we've seen, in Tantric sex there is one mind, one body, and one spirit shared between lovers. Passion is built not only on physical sensation but on the intimacy of oneness, on the knowledge that loving another is also self-love and that merging with another is to become part of the stream of life, past, present, and future.

Good sex need not become routinized, need not seem a chore, need not become a fantasy to be found in the arms of someone other than your present partner. Every sexual union can become more fulfilling, even more a combining of physical and spiritual love than the last.

Passion for sex translates into passion for life—and vice versa. You cannot be passionate about life if you do not see its beauty and the beauty of the world around you. Without a sense of wonder and awe, sex and life are unfulfilling. Sex, of all human acts (and good human sex is quite different from sex between the lower animals, since human sex involves the mind as well as the body), is the best expression of the interconnectedness of all things on earth and in the universe. The union of two is the union of all.

Yet passion for life is impossible if you are not healthy, and you cannot be healthy without following the principles of a clean diet, balanced breath, and fluid movement. All work on both body and mind, all are geared to a steady flow of energy through the chakras, all are fundamental steps toward self-mastery.

The Tantric masters regulate their food based on time, quality, and quantity—just as you will. They eat foods that stimulate metabolism, not overload it—just as you will. They fast every night to make sure the body can do its metabolic work unimpeded—just as you will. They do not snack and they do not eat when they're not hungry—and neither will you. (Remember the times when you've fallen in love? I've interviewed more than five hundred women on this subject, and all—yes, all—reported that during those times food lost its importance. They were hungry for their partners.)

The Tantric masters pay attention to their breathing as well. They know that they can bring their entire autonomic nervous system into balance simply by controlling their breathing pattern. They know how to send breath directly to the various chakras—and by the time you finish this book, so will you.

The Tantric masters know, too, something only acknowledged in Western society in the past twenty-five years: that the body holds emotions within it in the form of physical blockages in various areas. Psychological stress—often unconsciously experienced—may lead to stiffness in the back or shoulders; anxiety will disturb the heart rate and close down the chest; anger at a loved one will cramp the pelvis. Movement is one means of unblocking the emotions and letting them flow freely into your consciousness, where they can be acknowledged and dealt with. I'm not surprised to see women sob on a treadmill. Great therapists like Ilana Rubenfeld can bring out emotions by manipulating the feet or backs of their patients. Yes, exercise will lead to a healthier body, but it will also lead to a healthier mind. As I say, the Tantric masters know how this works—and so will you.

———

Tantric union requires a clearing of the body and mind of everything that is not of the sexual moment—the psychological, spiritual, and wondrously physical pleasure of the sexual act itself. The Tantric master is a person who has mastered all aspects of the mental and spiritual self as well as his physical being. But we do not have to become Tantric masters ourselves to adopt Tantric principles to ensure our sexual vitality. We can begin the journey of self-mastery with the basic Tantric simplicities of diet, movement, and breathing.

It is important that we seek partners who are on the same journey; otherwise the achievement of Tantric union is a more difficult (though not impossible) task. With such partners, we will soon reach a fundamental goal: divine orgasm, the subject of the following chapter.

Chapter 7

*D*IVINE ORGASM

The physiology of a woman's orgasm is relatively simple. Stimulation of an erogenous zone (the lips, the ears, the inner thighs, the breasts, the vagina, the anus, the clitoris), either by oneself or by a partner, sends a signal to the brain that pleasure is on the way, and the brain, an adherent of pleasure, responds through the nervous system, which increases the blood flow and muscle tension in the genital area. The vagina becomes more lubricated, the clitoris swells. There is an increase in heart rate, blood pressure rises (causing the "sex flush" most women experience during intercourse), and assuming the woman feels safe, there are no distractions, and the partner is an experienced and able lover, orgasm occurs, resulting in contractions of the vaginal muscles and a general sense that there's no better physical feeling in the whole world.

The length of time an orgasm lasts varies from woman to woman. So does the ability to have multiple orgasms, the ability to control one's breath, the skill in controlling the inner vaginal muscles. In essence, however, all women go through the same biological processes, from arousal to climax to rest. (Men go through an identical cycle, the difference being that the physiological process involves different hormones.)

That's the physiology, but to me an orgasm isn't completely satisfying if it's purely physiological—if the mind and spirit of both partners aren't involved.

———

Tantra and Taoism both speak of a way to transform sexual energy into spiritual energy, individual ecstasy into the ecstasy of all life.

I should emphasize again that orgasm is not a goal of Tantric teaching; it is spoken of merely as one of the many means to self-mastery. In fact, Tantric training requires the conservation of orgasm, an act that itself requires a focusing of the mind, one of the steps in the process of enlightenment. Pleasure is not its goal; spiritual union and enlightenment are. Orgasm from a Tantric perspective creates both emotional and physical attachment to another (or to the act itself), which makes it difficult for one to achieve enlightenment.

Although all the chakras are involved in orgasm, it is most closely related to the second and third. First we must create a flow, a function of the second chakra. Here is where we begin to become moist, as our bodies are stimulated. Foreplay causes the stimulation of the flow, which prepares the mucous membranes for activity. Then as we begin to get lubricated and "heat up," we move up the chakra ladder and the fire (third chakra) begins to burn. If the fire isn't burning properly, we won't achieve orgasm or the heightened experience of increased energy. During orgasm, we let go and open our hearts (fourth chakra). When cultivating sexual energy into spiritual energy we go much higher, up to the seventh chakra, the realm of enlightenment. At this point, the sexual energy of a man and a woman is transformed into superpotency, and the kundalini—the dominant force in the human body—is started on its upward flow from the pelvis through the heart to the brain, from which it ascends to the realm of spirituality.

Because our hearts and brains as well as our genitals are engaged in Tantric sex, you can see why a partner is so impor-

CHAKRA (SANSKRIT)	MEANING NAME	ELEMENT
One (Muladhara)	Root/support	Earth
Two (Svadhisthana)	Sweetness	Water
Three (Manipura)	Lustrous jewel	Fire
Four (Anahata)	Unstruck	Air
Five (Visshudha)	Purification	Ether
Six (Ajna)	To perceive	Light
Seven (Sahasrara)	Thousandfold	?

tant to orgasm. Physically, a woman can have as intense an orgasm through masturbation as she can with a partner (it requires mastery of the PC muscle, a subject I'll take up later in the book), but *spiritually* a partner is necessary, whether of the same or the opposite sex.

Having said that, though, I'm still in favor of masturbation *if* it helps women come in contact with their own sexual bodies, or simply as a means to release sexual tension. In today's climate, where casual sex can be downright dangerous, a single woman can be without a partner for a long time, especially if she wants to wait for someone she really clicks with. In such cases, masturbation is definitely advised. (Actually, some 33 percent of my clients never masturbate. Many don't even want to talk about their genitals. Maybe it's because girls, unlike boys, really don't have much to compare with one another.) But even if you have a partner, masturbation can be an aid toward learning how to control orgasm. It does not deplete sexual energy in women as it does in men. And it's pleasurable!

But don't overdo it. It may cause you to lose sensitivity in the genital area (I'm against vibrators and dildos, by the way, because they also cause a loss of sensitivity), and while fantasy may be involved, there is no spiritual union in the act. Mutual love involves the body, the mind, and the soul.

In Tantra women are to be worshiped by men. They are to be satisfied on all levels. For them particularly, sexuality is more than the merging of genitalia; it involves mind and spirit as well. Women's sexual energy is involved in giving but more involved in receiving, for it is we who create other humans. Several ancient texts claim that sex is more important to a woman than it is to a man. (Modern medicine bears this out. It has found that male pheromones, absorbed by a woman into her system during the sex act, help regulate her fertility and ensure the health of her reproductive system. Regular sexual intercourse, as we've seen, keeps our vaginas lubricated and improves our overall well-being.)

During Tantric union, every aspect of the sexual act transforms ordinary awareness into enlightened vision. The man sees the woman as a deity, her sexual organ as the throne of enlightenment, her sexual fluids as divine nectar. The woman, like the man, loses her ego to the union and is therefore able to transform passion into a state of meditative awareness, free from lust and ego involvement. According to the Tantric master Tsongkhapa, "The supreme female . . . practitioner . . . should be diligent and not lazy and should have a passion to practice and attain the spiritual attainments. Having found one like that," he advises men, "unite with her, do all the assorted ritual activities, and enjoy the pleasure of intense passion."

All faiths and philosophies, East and West, hold spiritual fulfillment as the greatest blessing we can experience. In the East, only a few—Tantric masters, Zen masters, fakirs—are apt to find it, since they are the ones who spend their lives searching for it. Most Westerners believe, however, that the search itself is folly, that spirituality is bestowed only through an unstinting obedience to God. Trying to "find" grace, as trying to "find" yourself, is ultimately an act of narcissism, a way of becoming insular, a descent from One to one.

To me, sex is union, giving and receiving. I believe it can be mastered, and that practice is essential. The more you love your partner, the better the sex will be, for you will engage your spiritual self as well as your physical one. Sex is not in itself enlightenment, but it is one of the great animal and spiritual forces of mankind—something done by all creatures. However, humans alone are capable of seeing the role of the spiritual in the act of love.

In my view, erotic sex is possible without ever achieving orgasm. The closeness, intimacy, and pleasure of caressing and being caressed by someone you love is to me far more rewarding than the spasm itself. And it is possible, metaphorically at least, to have an orgasmic experience without having sex. According to therapist Rose Marie Raccioppi, orgasm is "the experience of the bliss of creation," and athletes and artists (among others) speak of it in connection with their work, not their genitals.

———

Unsatisfactory sex is the cause of much disease among women. If a woman's partner fails to satisfy her, she will not receive essential nutrients from him. Sexual frustration creates anger, and the pungency of anger imbalances a woman's sexual organs and blood.

Physiological and psychological problems can also hinder the enjoyment or even the practice of sex. If you have a problem with blood pressure, for example, you may have trouble achieving orgasm because you don't get sufficient blood to the genitals. If you are anxiety-ridden, your mind will be distracted and you won't be able to focus on the sex act or even on your own enjoyment. If your genital muscles—and particularly your pubococcygeus muscle, the one that contracts during orgasm—are weak, you can't fully experience the delicious contractions of climax. If you're stressed, if you have an incapacitating disease, if your stomach is too full, if you have a cold or a headache, if you're angry or sad—all these will rob you of sexual pleasure. So deeply is sex dependent on freedom of the body and mind that any glitch will throw it off. Many women have told me that to enjoy sex, they have to "break through a wall," the physical and mental distractions that inhibit freedom of the body, and unfocus the mind. It can take time to free the mind and relax the body. Hence the value of foreplay and the advantage of a tender and experienced lover.

There is no question, therefore, that orgasm depends on a healthy body and a healthy mind. To return to my primary sphere, the physical, it's obvious that good sex is based on endurance, muscle function, and good blood circulation. Practice helps. Stamina helps. Continued exercise is essential.

During orgasm, the tendency of a woman's body, like a man's, is to release energy outward. This generally goes unnoticed, since the release is not so clearly apparent in a woman, and patently during each female orgasm less energy is lost than with a man. Nevertheless, if a woman learns to draw her energy inward and upward, using her muscles and her mind, she will heighten her sexual experience. Instead of an orgasm discharging, say, one hundred volts of energy, it will charge (not discharge) one hundred thousand volts throughout the body. Quite a difference! To effect it we must work on the pubococ-

Four Steps to a Fulfilled Relationship

- *Make each day as if it is your first encounter*
- *Accept your relationship as a gift*
- *Choose someone who is compatible*
- *Practice the art of committing to one partner*

cygeus muscle—as noted, the one that expands and contracts during orgasm. (The PC muscle was "discovered" by Dr. Arnold Kegel, who realized its importance in childbirth and incontinence. Only later did we "dare" to speak of it in connection with sex.)

You'll see what muscle I'm talking about if the next time you urinate you consciously stop the urine from flowing. The muscle you use to do this is the PC muscle. If you exercise it regularly, you'll find your orgasms will become more intense and, as a "by-benefit," as you age your chances of incontinence will decrease and your vagina will remain tight. Indeed, female Tantric masters reportedly have such control over their PC muscles that they are able to prevent entry of the penis at will.

A client named Kathy told me that two years earlier a physician had recommended that she surgically have her PC muscle tightened so she and her husband could enjoy sex more, and that she'd had the operation.

"What exercises did he recommend in conjunction with the operation?" I asked.

She looked at me blankly. "Exercises?"

If the doctor had been standing with her, I'd have asked him if he wanted his testicles sewn up so they wouldn't hang!

The PC muscle can be exercised daily without engaging in intercourse. Leg lifts are particularly helpful. You'll find specific exercises later in this book, but as a start sit on a chair with a pillow or rolled-up towel under your tailbone. Take a deep breath. On exhalation, draw up the muscles as if you are stopping urination, and then release. Repeat this ten times.

When you've practiced the exercise and feel yourself proficient at it, try the same contraction and release when you masturbate (you can do the chair exercise in public, but I'd recommend privacy for the masturbatory one). Again, once you've achieved proficiency—if your orgasms seem more powerful—adopt the technique for sexual intercourse. My client

Janet had always relied on clitoral stimulation to achieve orgasm. Once she learned to use her PC muscle, she told me that she felt as if she was having sex for the first time. In fact, in a profound way, she was!

Note that breathing is as important as exercise in developing control over the PC muscle. Sandy, who was adept at both, felt herself getting so lubricated during exercise class that she became embarrassed. She wanted to know if there was anything wrong with her because she'd begun to feel new sensations throughout her body. I assured her that there was nothing wrong—and much right. "With your new glow," I told her, "you'll find a partner soon. Time to take those exercises one step further."

When a woman learns metabolic breathing and combines it with her PC muscle exercises, her orgasm can be prolonged and its intensity heightened. When she is beginning to feel the heat build toward orgasm, she should draw in the muscles of the pelvis and vagina and tighten the PC muscle. The muscle contractions must be accompanied by deep, steady breathing in order to leave time for inhalation. As the orgasm nears its peak, the woman keeps drawing the muscles inward toward the sensations, which will grow stronger and vibrate throughout the body, energizing all organ systems, even the brain. I'm not saying that you'll experience a "perfect" orgasm, or even feel an appreciable difference the first time you try the technique, but over time I guarantee increased sexual pleasure—and you'll enjoy practicing!

Nothing tones the pelvic area's muscles and ligaments better than an orgasm. Exercises for the PC muscle in conjunction with metabolic breathing are a close second. But for maximum orgasmic pleasure, the whole area—indeed, the whole body—must be flexible, limber, pliant, relaxed.

If you have chronic lower-back pain, the last thing you think of is the pleasure you'll receive from orgasmic contractions—quite the contrary. Often our posture indicates issues of control (people who walk with a stoop feel they lack the support they need), and bad posture often leads to lower-back problems. Our posture also indicates how comfortable we are with our sexuality. Many women who are inhibited sexually lock their hips and walk with their pelvis tilted back. But when the hips are locked, energy stagnates. There's no way to stimulate the second and third chakras, no way you can experience the vibrations of the pelvic area that occur during orgasm.

Stand up for a minute and swing your hips from side to side, then do a few circles in each direction. How does it make you feel? Restricted? If so, you may feel restricted during orgasm.

Annie came to me with lower-back pain. She walked with her pelvis tilted back and did not have good hip rotation. She did not initially talk of her lack of interest in sex or the quality of her orgasms, but over time, working with me on opening her hips and learning to rotate her pelvis, she was able to discuss the issues that discouraged her sexual interest. These problems were not deep-seated, they simply needed expression. She, like many women, had been brought up to think that her sexual function was to satisfy her man, taking her own pleasure "as best she can." She also believed that her ability to achieve orgasm would decrease as she got older.

This is the exact opposite of Tantric teaching. Our lack of understanding of the pleasure we can derive from sex, and our unwillingness to do the routine exercises that will increase sexual pleasure at any age, is a great misfortune.

———

Can you eat your way to sexual potency? Not really. It's true that many so-called aphrodisiacs are rich in nutrients that support sexual function (although the most famous, Spanish fly, simply irritates the urinary tract, causing a reaction that is felt as "heat"—though it's hardly sexual heat), but as noted earlier, one woman's aphrodisiac is merely another's bird's nest soup.

Actually, many sensual foods are themselves sexual organs—

tomatoes and all seed-containing fruits, as well as eggs of all kinds, including caviar—in the animal kingdom. Remember, too, that flowers are the sexual organs of plants, fruits their ovaries. Some sensual foods simply *look* sexy—asparagus, for example, or bananas, artichokes, and avocados, with the added plus that all are nutrient rich.

I know a woman named Susan who, when she wants to get her husband and herself aroused, prepares sautéed asparagus with lemon and drippings of butter, honey-ginger glazed shrimp, and pomegranates. When Eastern philosophers speak of food in relation to sex, they say that the food must be light, moist, and sweet—just like the meal Susan prepares for her husband.

"Lightness" refers to those foods that are easily digested. Most fruits, for example, take only twenty minutes to digest. Some vegetables—leeks, onions, squash, artichokes, asparagus, and mushrooms among them—are also quickly assimilated into the bloodstream. Fruit juice and vegetable juice cocktails are the most easily digested.

"Moist" foods are those that provide lubrication to our tissues. Since to achieve orgasm the body must secrete fluids, it makes sense that the more fluids available, the easier it will be to come to climax. Honey, melons, avocados, fresh figs, squash, shrimp, almonds, and sea vegetables belong in this category.

By "sweet" foods, I *don't* mean cookies, cakes, or foods laced with sugar. I'm talking about the natural sugars found in fruits, vegetables, and legumes. These foods provide the energy and stamina needed for muscle contractions, though if taken in excess, they overstimulate and fatigue the body by depleting the adrenals. Orgasm itself is "sweet," too, in that it's pleasurable and wonderful. My observations have shown that when we have the sweetness of sex in our lives, we don't require as much sweet food in our diets.

While no scientific study has ever been done on the relation of food to female orgasm (studies *have* been done on the relation of food to men's ability to achieve erection), it has been postulated that men and women who cannot reach orgasm are sometimes aided by supplements of the vitamin niacin (which releases the histamines stored in the body that are essential for achieving orgasm), particularly when taken along with folic acid and vitamin B6 (vitamin B6 decreases prolactin levels, which in turn may increase libido). And calcium and vitamin B5 have been cited as helping to increase sexual stamina. But vitamins are not enough. Sexual organs feed off nutrients—they are the last to be supplied by the body—so it's obvious that a healthy diet is essential for good sex. One of my patients experienced a remarkable increase in sexual desire and pleasure simply by getting off refined candies and cookies (substitutes for sex on many levels) while keeping the rest of her diet the same. Women find themselves eating desserts when what they really need is to have sex. And diet affects the mind. The feeling of "not being in the mood" may be related not only to too much food but also to an improper balance of different kinds of food.

Veronica, a young-looking fifty-three, was constantly fatigued and depressed. This was "normal," she was told, due to hormonal changes common at her age. Although she continued to engage in sex to satisfy her lover, she was faking orgasm and bringing him to ejaculation as quickly as possible so that she did not have to deal with the vaginal irritation caused by lack of lubrication.

Her diet consisted of muffins and coffee in the morning (coffee, she explained, gave her a "boost"), a bagel at lunch, pasta for dinner when she ate out, and a mixture of noodles and vegetables from a salad bar when she dined at home. Often she would grab a nonfat yogurt to satisfy her craving for sweets.

Veronica was depleting her system of nutrients. It could muster energy only to keep her metabolism functioning—there was nothing left over for sex. She needed nutrient-dense foods, so I suggested those that would get her hormones flowing again and lubricate her cells, foods rich in omega-3 fatty acids like tuna, mackerel, and salmon that she should substitute for pasta on the nights she went out for dinner. When she did choose pasta, I recommended that she sprinkle it with ground flaxseeds from the health-food store. Next, she changed her snacks to fruits, pumpkin seeds, and sunflower seeds. I also suggested that she choose bean mixtures and cooked greens on the nights she bought dinner at the salad bar, or at least add alfalfa sprouts to her raw salads. Finally, I advised her to take a vitamin-mineral supplement that contained at least 400 IU of vitamin E. Within ten days, her fatigue levels had diminished. By the fifth week, her nights, she told me, were "interesting again."

———

While not aphrodisiacs, here is a list of foods containing the necessary ingredients for sexual potency:

Figs
Asparagus
Avocados
Honey
Artichokes
Tomatoes
Leeks and onions
Shrimp
Almond milk
Seaweed

Obviously, even if you eat them all, you won't necessarily increase your sexual pleasure or the power of your orgasm—too many other factors are involved—but they do provide a ground-work for sexual satisfaction—and they taste good. Others have found that nuts, seeds, grains, alfalfa seeds or sprouts, and many leafy greens, which contain nutrients used to synthesize dopamine and acetylcholine, stimulate sexual pleasure.

Some foods also *smell* good, and a woman's sense of smell, far more than a man's, is deeply involved in sexual pleasure. The herb rosemary added to a meal will heighten that sense, and there are many forms of incense and perfume that can be a wonderful accompaniment to making love.

Indeed, all the senses are involved in sex, for all send messages to the brain. And the brain, as we'll see in the next chapter, is as important to sex as the heart and the genitals.

$\mathcal{T}$HE MIND-BODY RESPONSE

Every time Jenny thinks about money, her lower back tenses and sex is painful. When Beth is angry at her husband but nevertheless has sex with him, she experiences trouble in her urinary tract. Anne's repressed sexual desire clearly leads to yeast infections.

By now it's no secret that the body and mind are closely linked, and nowhere is this more evident than when it comes to sex. One of the fundamental joys of orgasm is the fact that the mind "lets go." If we're distracted, the sex isn't good.

Indeed, your body is the manifestation of your thoughts. Anxiety often manifests itself in the neck and shoulders. If you're upset, your stomach secretes acid; when you're afraid, there's a rush of adrenaline. Rita, one of my clients, was chronically constipated, and we were able to figure out why only when she described how unhappy she was that her mother had moved into a nursing home.

In order to experience love, we need not only to love ourselves but also to keep our minds focused on our partner. Personally, I don't fantasize during sex, and thinking of things other than sex when you're making love is one of the great deterrents to sexual intimacy. Almost as bad is concentrating solely on your own pleasure without regard to your partner. When I find myself thinking, What about how *I* feel?, I know I'll have to choose another lover. If I can think about him, then he can think about me! Diversions and distractions are experienced first in the mind, then transmitted to the body, which can turn off sex as easily as the hand can turn off a television set.

A friend of mine told me she had to split with her lover because he had a mole on his penis. "Every time we make love," she said, "even if we make love in the dark, I *see* it. It's ugly. I just can't get over the thought of it."

He volunteered to have it surgically removed, but it was too late. "I'd still imagine it as being there," she told me. "Seeing a *different* penis would be just as much a turn-off."

Whether their sexual incompatibility was a psychological problem of hers or a physical one of his (he had no such trouble with previous lovers) is immaterial. The point is that her mind got in the way and she was unable to free it. Other women have told me that they can't stop thinking of their lovers with other women, real or imagined.

Freeing the mind from all thoughts except those of sex is the essence of sexual pleasure. This would seem obvious—Eastern philosophers speak of the "one-pointed mind" and Tantric teaching explains that sexual adepts can remove their minds from their environments—but it is often the *unconscious* mind that prevents us from experiencing sexual freedom. We are bound by our parents' teachings, our guilts, our secrets.

There is no one less sexually inhibited than a young child, unashamed of nakedness, publicly masturbating, proud of body and unchecked in mind. How quickly that freedom vanishes! "Don't touch yourself." "*Peepee*'s a bad word." "Put on some clothes." "Don't look at Daddy naked." The list of prohibitions grows quickly, and so by the time we get to school, "bathroom words" are giggled at with our peers, games like "doctor" are played routinely in secret, and our natural curiosity is deemed prurient, bad, unhealthy.

When I was seven, my teacher mentioned a book called *Pippie Longstocking.* I burst out in embarrassed laughter and was too shy to explain why. In fact, *pippie* was my aunt's word for penis, and when I went home that night, I blurted out to my mother that my teacher had said a dirty word.

Adults who are sexually ignorant (in my experience, a greater number than one might think) put taboos on sex and the sexual organs. A girl of seven, playing on her uncle's lap, was reprimanded by her mother. "It's not nice to straddle like that. People will think you're a bad girl." Another was told to cross her legs because it wasn't "ladylike" to show her knees. (Imagine the effect on the second chakra!)

But it isn't only faulty sexual instruction that can inhibit us. A male friend of mine went through two years of impotence because he'd been having an affair when his wife died suddenly of cancer and he assumed the guilt for her death. A woman raped in a subway station has not had an orgasm since. Another molested by her stepfather entered into dozens of affairs without pleasure and without release.

By the time we become adults, we often have lost faith in our sexual bodies. Many women don't like to get undressed in front of their lovers because they don't like certain parts of their bodies, such as their thighs. Once when I undressed, my lover announced that he hadn't thought my legs were so big. A different lover complained that my breasts were too small. I became paranoid about my thighs, overexercising them to the point of idiotic fatigue. And my breasts lost their sensitivity for five years, regaining it only with my present lover, who thinks small, firm athletic breasts are spectacular.

We are most vulnerable during sex because we have to be unguarded to experience heightened sexual pleasure with another human being. The fewer our inhibitions, the more open we can become, and the more willingly and freely we can give ourselves to another (and he can give himself to us). That is why sex is best with someone you love—but also why, with nothing psychic to gain or lose, sex with a relative stranger sometimes can be so arousing and physically fulfilling. Still, unresolved emotional issues can get in the way of sex with someone you love. By keeping the mind focused—with no emotional, professional, or environmental distractions—sex becomes the optimum expression of love, of oneself and the other.

The mind is a complicated, as yet unfathomable organ. If we could *actually* train it, we would undoubtedly be healthier and there would be fewer of us with inadequate sex lives no matter the childhood inhibitions or adult traumas.

For now, though, we must only do the best we can, recognizing that there is a direct connection between mind and body in virtually all spheres of life, that the body contains emotions that can only be released physically (the pioneering work of Wilhelm Reich and Ilana Rubenfeld has proven this), and that physical well-being is essential to mental health.

And the link between body and mind is breath.

———

According to ancient yoga tradition, we are encased in five sheaths—the body, energy, and three dimensions of the mind. We have already seen that through breath we can fathom the subtleties of the body sheath and the pranic sheath; we can do the same with the mind.

When we modulate breath, we can have access to the patterns of the mind. In fact, the rhythm of breath is the most obvious physical indication of a person's emotional or mental health. When I get a call from a new client, for example, I can almost always determine the state of her mind not by listening to her words but by listening to the way she breathes.

The body is the physical manifestation of the mind. When we change our thoughts, our body responds. Thoughts can be changed by changing breathing patterns; modulating breathing patterns can heighten concentration and, when it comes to sex, pleasure.

But breathing is something almost all of us do unconsciously. You may be aware of your own breath now because you're reading about it, but you won't be when you're at work or in the middle of watching a movie. Indeed, I'm not asking you to be conscious of your breath all the time; I'm only saying that through *conscious breath* you can begin to change many physical and emotional aspects of yourself.

The strength of your breathing relates to everything that you think or do. The less you fully use your lungs, the weaker your physical strength becomes, thus adversely affecting your entire metabolism. We've seen that rapid shallow chest breathing is synonymous with acute states of anxiety, and we know that sighing (pausing after exhalation) is a characteristic of depression. When we are angry or about to cry, we hold our breath after an inhalation.

Breath is connected to the mind. Left-nostril dominance is associated with right-brain activities; right-nostril dominance is associated with left-brain activities. Jerks in the flow of breath indicate jerkiness in the thought process, as the mind hops distractedly from one thought to another. Breathing irregularities also express irregularities in the stream of thought. Pauses in breath intensify emotional states, and shallow breathing deenergizes both body and mind, numbing awareness. As noted, if you are conscious of your breath, you can change your mental and physical states.

Start by becoming aware of the flow of breath through your nostrils. This allows you to become aware of both your inner and outer environments, the mind-body interaction. Is your left more active than your right, or vice versa? Every 90 to 120 minutes, the nostrils switch dominance, but overall one nostril or the other will be dominant most of the time (this varies from person to person). For example, suppose your left nostril is most active and you decide to do some exercise. Chances are that the right will dominate within a few minutes.

You can feel your nostrils switch with this simple exercise: Breathe through each nostril holding the other one closed to see which is more open. Suppose you find it is the left. Lie down on your left side and pay attention to the right nostril. It will automatically become active within ten minutes.

Ideally, if you are balanced, your right nostril is dominant when:

You're physically active.
Your body is warm.
You're hungry.
You're eating.
You're engaging in short-term, intense effort.

And your left nostril is dominant when:

You're quiet, at rest.
Your body is cool.
You're thirsty.
You're drinking liquids.
You're engaging in long-term, sustained effort.

It is said that during sexual intercourse the male should have the right nostril dominant, the woman the left. This makes sense, since the female is usually more the receiver, the male the more aggressive. (I'm not saying that the woman can't or shouldn't initiate sex, but even when that's the case, it's often the man who *becomes* the more active.) When you pay attention to your breath while making love, you'll be amazed at how quickly you'll become aware of not only your own rhythm but your partner's. In so doing, you'll be forced to pay attention to your immediate environment, free of distractions, and soon you

MIND/BODY BALANCE

BREATH
INHALATION – EXHALATION

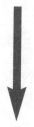

AUTONOMIC NERVOUS
SYSTEM RESPONSE

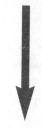

MIND 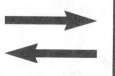 BODY

and your partner will develop a rhythm that will lead to intense mutual satisfaction.

In essence, the rhythm of breath and the rhythm of sex should be the same. Tantric masters believe that the circulation of prana is most balanced when the female's left nostril is dominant and the male's right. If you're face-to-face, all chakras are aligned, and modulating your breath will cause a harmonious vibrancy for both partners—a very powerful and stimulating union. If, on the other hand, you're breathing from the chest and he from the diaphragm, you may achieve orgasm, but that's all.

David, my current lover, is my best because we've learned to balance our breathing, and thus balance our bodies and our minds and enjoy each other's vibrations and rhythms. Mind open to sensation but closed to everything else, breathing in harmony, one with each other, excited yet at peace—there is no better sensation in the world. It is the sensation of love.

———

Breathing has another sexual function: It lets you smell. To me, there is no better smell than the body of my lover, but others use perfume, incense, or flowers to heighten their sexual enjoyment. The sense of smell, of course, varies from person to person; what smells good to one can turn off another. The nose, through its terminal, the brain, is capable of distinguishing among thousands of specific odors. Remember: The limbic system is the seat of our emotions, and our olfactory bulbs—those organs responsible for smell—are directly connected to it. That's why smell can elicit such an emotional response. Along with touch, smell is our most primitive sense (it is the dominant one in many mammals), and in all of us it is loaded with instinctive associations, perhaps originating millions of years ago.

The relationship between smell and the mind has been recognized for millennia. Aromatic herbs and oils have been used as aphrodisiacs and seductive potions since the earliest civilizations. *Kyphi,* an ancient Egyptian perfume, was thought to infuse sleep with bright dreams. The Greeks used aromatic oils as antidepressants, to aid sleep, and as aphrodisiacs. Today, researchers have found that odors can and do influence mood, evoke emotions, counteract stress. Products from bathroom tissues to underarm deodorants are given smells, and we all know that the perfume industry grosses billions of dollars annually. Too, we don't generally wear perfume just to smell good, at least when we put it on our neck or between our breasts. We use it as a sexual lure.

My favorite example of how an odor works concerns a client appropriately named May, a woman of thirty-one. She came to me complaining of being overweight, although she seemed trim and fit.

"How do you *know* you're too heavy?" I asked.

"Because my husband doesn't want to make love to me."

"How many times a month do you have sex?"

"Once. And only because I insist."

Once a month was clearly not enough for this seemingly sexually radiant woman.

"What happens most nights?"

"He turns away when I try to embrace him."

Maybe it's how you smell, I thought—though she smelled fine to me. I gave her some diluted ylang-ylang and suggested she put it on her neck that night. It had a scent, I knew from personal experience, that could stimulate sexual desire. She tried it. It worked. She called me a few days later to ask where she could buy a bottle of it.

"Any health-food store or bath shop," I told her.

"I want to use it as a bath oil," she explained. "For both of us."

As we've seen, scents can unlock emotions. The smell of a flower can raise your spirits; our lover's body odor can add to our love or turn it off. Odors can affect our ability to concentrate, make us feel euphoric, get us sexually aroused. When we bathe or massage with essential oils, we absorb some of their chemical constituents. I find that using oils of ylang-ylang with neroli and sandlewood in my bath eases stress. Baths of juniper, bergamot, and lavender also relax me, especially after a workout. And rosemary, which has become my perfume, makes me feel confident. Don't ask me why. It's all in the smell.

———

Food affects the mind as well as the body. In Ayurvedic nutrition, there are three kinds of foods that affect the mind:

Tamasic foods: These dull the mind, produce inertia, produce what I call a "carbohydrate stupor," and are generally hard to digest. Processed meats (not available when the Ayurvedic texts were written, but never mind), fats, most cheeses, fried foods, heavy sweets, and cooked beef, chicken, and fowl fall into this category.

Rajasic foods: These produce energy, speed up the metabolism, and stimulate the mind. They include pepper, ginger, hot spices, onions, coffee, canned sweetened fruits, and fruit juices. Taken in moderation, they will aid digestion as well as the mind. Overuse them, and you'll be running at too fast a speed, and clear thinking will suddenly become fuzzy.

Sattvic foods: These produce clarity, harmony, and balance in the mind. Almost all vegetables and fruits are in this category, including artichokes, asparagus, dates, ghee, berries, and figs. Honey, too, is a sattvic food.

Most people's diets—mine, too—include all three. In my experience, strict vegetarians (those eating predominantly sattvic foods) are indeed calmer than the average person, but I like a little spice and passion in my life, and there's no question that at some dinners a chocolate cake is preferable to a discussion of the philosophy of Nietzsche. All rhubarb and no ginger make Jill a dull girl.

Just as food can influence mind, so can mind influence what foods we eat. At one of my recent lectures, I was talking about the benefits of the nighttime fast. A woman raised her hand.

"What do I do when I want something crunchy and munchy at eleven P.M.?" she asked. Her tone and manner suggested that she was edgy and that the answer was important to her.

"What's your normal diet?" I asked.

"A little meat and a lot of salad."

"Cookies? Candies? Potato chips?"

"No way. My husband wants me to stay thin."

"And you?"

Her voice became defiant. "I want to stay thin, too."

"Then why," I asked, "are you so angry?"

Her face turned red and she gave a little gasp, as though I had penetrated some intimate secret. Quickly, she sat down.

I felt bad about embarrassing her—I had not counted on so intense a response—yet it gave me a chance to explain.

When we're angry, I told the group, we often crave crunchy foods. Eating them satisfies the feeling of wanting to bite someone's head off. Similarly, when we're depressed, or feeling unworthy or unattractive, we crave sweet, soft foods containing fats and carbohydrates—"comfort foods," as my mother calls them.

"What do you find yourself craving when you're with your lover or are feeling in love?"

A different woman answered: "Who craves food?"

I smiled. "Exactly."

I never got to work with the angry woman—she was almost surely now angry at *me*—but if I had, I would have suggested she include some grains in her diet to give her sweetness and I would have limited all rajasic foods. The last thing she needed was to exacerbate her anger through her diet.

In *Ayurvedic Healing: A Comprehensive Guide,* Dr. David Frawley says, "Emotions have the same effect [on our bodies] as foods or herbs of the same energetic quality. Anger can damage the liver as much as alcoholism. So herbs and diet are not enough if the taste of the mind has not changed." He has made up a list of the six tastes and their corresponding emotions.

Sweet—love
Salty—greed
Sour—envy
Pungent—hatred
Bitter—grief
Astringent—fear

Obviously, the physical/emotional cravings we have for certain tastes are so strong that the simple question "Why don't we change our diet and simply eat wholesome foods?" is answered by the fact that we are pulled by our emotions—and by our tastes. In other words, it isn't as easy as it sounds.

From a biochemical perspective, our blood-sugar level is one of the biggest contributors to our moods—and to our sexual radiance.

When we have a steady supply of glucose in our bloodstream, we don't have radical shifts in mood or energy levels. Do you get moody at certain times of the day? If so, most likely you've had a drop in your blood-sugar level. A glass of diluted grape juice will fix things instead of the four P.M. candy bar or frozen yogurt. And blood sugar is the reason for eating oatmeal in the morning instead of a sugary cereal, which may make you produce too much insulin and experience a quick drop in energy after eating it. Oatmeal (with a fresh-fruit topping if you want) takes longer to digest, and you'll get a steady flow of insulin as the digestive process works. The result is that the glucose level is constant, and your mind and body will stay alert (though since it's the morning, probably for work, alas, rather than sex).

———

All animals share the same primal urges for food, sleep, self-preservation, and sex. Only humans, though, can regulate these urges consciously, and so become free to experience higher levels of consciousness. This is a basic tenet of Eastern philosophy, and the Tantric master will have overcome all primitive urges to devote his bodily, mental, and spiritual life to enlightenment.

The vast majority of us, however, will be constrained to some degree by our primal urges. When it comes to sex, the more we can include the spiritual element, the more satisfying it will be.

If we think of sex—and enjoy sex—simply as a physical act, it soon becomes routinized. That's one of the reasons there's so much infidelity. But if we can make sex different every time, even with the same partner—if we can experience it in the moment, with our minds directed only to giving and receiving pleasure—then each sexual union will be new and different.

Sexual intercourse is an exchange of energy that has the potential of uniting us with another human being to create a new life. Either subconsciously or consciously we're all aware of this; that's why we are attracted to sex in the first place. (That it feels good is simply a nature-given by-product, a kind of come-on for procreation.) But when it's denied, both our minds and our bodies lose energy and look for compensation. In the case of women, too often that compensation is food.

When we lose the passion for love, we tend to sublimate. We're depressed and feel unworthy, and so we turn to tasmic foods (you don't see sexually vital people walking along eating a doughnut). Excess weight is often a sign of low self-esteem, frequently caused by an unhappy sexual relationship. If we've had a bad time with a lover, we are sometimes fearful of a new relationship, and so we eat to (generally unconsciously) create a barrier between ourselves and potential lovers.

This happened with Lisa, an attractive woman who came to me after getting out of a bad relationship and gaining twenty-five pounds by eating at night. Her weight gain was, of course, the physical manifestation of something that was going on in her mind—she didn't *want* to be attractive; it was too dangerous.

Once we located her fear of being unloved, we were able to address her weight. I had her substitute exercise for food at night, followed by a hot bath of essential oils. I also gave her a flower essence formula that worked on her mind to help increase her self-confidence and eliminate her self-doubt. I told her to visualize herself as a female warrior, and that every time she felt unsafe she should think of how strong and vibrant she was. It took a month of continual work, but when she began to shed pounds, she was able to look more closely at her mind and recognize what had happened. It's possible to change physical habits created by the mind if we become aware of their origin.

Nobody stays on an even keel; all of us have psychological ups and downs throughout our lives. My own weight has fluctuated as my relationships and my self-esteem have changed. Early on I might have had more trouble recognizing my mental problems if it had not been for Julie.

Julie came to me when I was in graduate school and in the unfortunate affair I described in the Introduction. She, on the other hand, described her own affair as "the most wonderful relationship imaginable."

"What makes it so wonderful?" I asked grouchily (and enviously).

"The sex. The intimacy. When we make love, I feel that I take on his personality and he takes mine. That we're one person, not two. I'm not only growing sexually, I'm growing spiritually."

Since I was already interested in diet—and was putting on weight as fast as I could—I asked about Julie's eating habits.

"Pasta every night," she said. "We meet in the Village, have our pasta, a salad, then walk home. By the time we get there, the food's digested and we're ready for sex."

Well, good for you, I thought, wishing she'd get out of my life. But in six months she returned, quite changed.

Seems that her ideal boyfriend had a drinking problem (too much wine with the pasta? I wondered) and they had split up.

Julie had ballooned from 108 pounds to 140; indeed, we were almost twins. Instead of trying to find a new man, she was filling her need for intimacy with food, but of course it didn't work. She had never felt so sad, so unworthy, she told me.

My heart went out to her. Her own problems so mirrored mine that I could see in her what I was unable to recognize in myself: By trying to pacify sadness and rejection with food, we were actually increasing the intensity of those emotions. By mistreating our bodies, we were mistreating our minds.

Shortly thereafter, I moved to Cleveland and Case Western Reserve to begin my Ph.D. studies, images of Julie—and myself—vivid in my brain.

———

Before I turn to my actual program, I want to mention two other sex-and-food issues, binges and stress.

I've talked about cravings earlier, and how they often reflect our emotional needs. Binges do the same thing, in a somewhat different fashion.

Irene binged. She would starve herself for days. ("No sugar," she proclaimed. "No fats. No flour products. No milk. No . . . No . . ."—you get the picture.) Then she would eat two boxes of cookies, a pint of sherbet, and three bagels every day for a week, feel guilty, and deny herself nourishing food for weeks thereafter. She became despondent sexually, even though she loved her fiancé, and when she was bingeing, she would not have sex. Obviously, she both wanted and feared intimacy; the bingeing spoke of deep ambivalence about herself and her lover.

Strangely, bingeing is far more difficult to "cure" than cravings, for I believe it stems from deeper psychological roots. In Irene's case, though, we were lucky. We made great progress by allowing her soy milk with a bowl of oatmeal in the morning, topped with lots of berries. This gave her the sweet, comforting feeling she needed to avoid her urge to binge. In the afternoon or evening (depending on her dinner plans), she had stir-fry, with a concentrated source of protein either from fish, chicken, or tofu, along with plenty of rice and vegetables. Soon her binges stopped and she was able to feel sexy again. Indeed, she became so balanced in body and mind (her blood sugar was regulated; she felt confident in herself and her lover) that she was even able to initiate sex, something she had never been able to do before.

Bingeing and cravings can cause stress on both body and mind, and stress guarantees inferior sex or no sex at all. It's an insidious cycle. Unsatisfying sex makes you anxious about sex the next time, and the stress the anxiety causes about sexual performance takes your head away from the single-mindedness sex requires.

Stress is all created in the mind. In turn, our bodies take the beating. Stress is the message our mind gives to our body that danger exists. If we think we're going to be fired—stress. If we think we'll be late turning in a job or an assignment—stress. If we're fatigued by overexercising in an effort to get our weight down—stress. If we're in a difficult relationship—stress. If we think we can't perform sexually—stress. If we think *our partner* can't perform sexually—stress. If we're too tired, come home late, are preoccupied—sexual stress.

Stress prepares the body for a survival response, and while sometimes this is a great benefit (a car is heading directly at you in the wrong lane—stress), more often the mind is sending a misleading or unnecessary message, and what seems stressful is in fact better treated calmly.

Let's say you find out your lover is seeing someone else—stress! Or is it? If you look at it calmly, you might reflect that you weren't that crazy about the s.o.b. anyway, and now *you* have the opportunity for new adventures. (Granted, this is an extreme example.)

But the New Agers are right. If you're in the moment, if there is no future to worry about and no pain to reflect upon from the past, then stress is nonexistent. (Stephan Rechtschaffen's book *Timeshifting* contains an excellent treatise on stress reduction, sexual and otherwise.) In the moment of actual orgasm, *nobody* feels stressed, for there is only that moment, even if what has led up to it is stressful.

Barring orgasm, meditation—an exercise for the mind—is a fine means of reducing stress, and sex itself can be made into a meditation or act of worship, as is the focus of Tantric sex. Indeed, until you can convert your sexual experiences into meditations, when your mind is single-pointed and all your senses are employed in service of the attainment of one ecstatic goal, you will always be tempted to search for new partners to fulfill your longings, and never be able to locate the total sense of satisfaction that ordinary sex hints at but cannot achieve.

Peggy and her fiancé, Greg, led stressful lives. They were both actors and their hours were sporadic. When one was working, the other was idle; when one was frenzied, the other was calm. They came to see me for nutritional advice—they needed to look good and maintain their weight and youthful appearance. But I saw at once that they were not communicating well, and I felt they would soon lose interest in each other.

I asked them about sex. They said it was "okay when [they] had time for it." They explained that often they didn't get home until very late and had too many things on their minds. Or that one wanted to be intimate when the other didn't. I recommended that they take one night each week and make a specific time to have sex, a time that *could not* be delayed or canceled. I told them to schedule this time as they would work or exercise. This would free up their minds at other times, but when they were together on the "date," they could think about, talk about, *experience* nothing but sex, his and hers for both of them. It was nothing more than an application of the Tantric principles of meditation and self-surrender, but it would, I explained, make their minds one-pointed.

They went away intrigued, and Greg called me two weeks later to leave a message. It was, simply, "Thank you."

I've covered the biochemical and philosophical ingredients for radiant sex. It's time now to turn specifically to the three elements—diet, breathing, and exercise—that will make it happen.

Part III

—

$\mathscr{A}$ TOTAL PROGRAM
FOR
SEXUAL RADIANCE

Chapter 9

*T*HE VITALITY DIET

In a nation in which a television commercial advises you to take an antacid *before* you eat dinner, it's small wonder the antidote to being overweight is often as pernicious as overeating: diets that starve you, promise "miracles," guarantee weight reduction in a week, give you a "full meal in a can."

But there are no miracles, no shortcuts, and getting thinner does not necessarily mean getting healthier. In my program, losing weight is secondary to gaining health. Vitality is the goal, not the shedding of pounds.

My vitality diet emphasizes flexibility with food on the theory that you can't be sexually flexible if you're not "food flexible." The recipes are nutritionally sound and delicious, but don't hesitate to experiment with other ingredients—on the theory that you can learn to experiment sexually if you learn to experiment with food.

I've included many spices and herbs; if you find new ones, try them—and write me about their effects. You're not expected to give up your old food friends. Just eat them at noon when your metabolism burns hottest. (I know that sometimes you'll "sin" even at night, and that sometimes you'll overeat. What's important is to follow the diet as a general rule.) My diet will allow you to derive maximum benefits from the foods you eat with the most efficient utilization of calories if you follow it most of the time.

I recognize that everyone is unique and that your diet is in many ways more personal than your religion. You will learn to balance your diet without copying anyone else's—and you'll discover that once you're on it, your sex life, too, will be totally individual and right for you alone. Best of all, your improved sex life will be different from what it was in the past. Our bodies are our own, and what we put into them, and how we use them, must pertain to our own distinctly personal biological requirements.

In broad terms, here's what I consider an ideal diet:

Upon arising: A sexual rejuvenator.

Breakfast: Fruit juice, fruit, toasted oats, soy milk, green tea, bancha tea, or kukicha tea. *Menopausal women will particularly benefit from soy milk on oats.*

Lunch: *Anything goes!* If you're starting the program, include your "comfort" foods, but be sure you eat cooked vegetables, especially the green leafy ones. Add grains—pasta, rice, or bread. As a protein source, focus on those of vegetable origins like beans and tofu (though if you crave meat, eat it in moderation—accompanied by vegetables). For a beverage with antioxidants, green tea.

Dinner: Mixed vegetables, rice, salad. The addition of a fish like sole (four ounces or so) is fine. Stay away from refined carbohydrates.

Snacks: Fresh fruits, fresh juices, and herbal teas between meals.

Supplements: Herbs, flower essences, vitamins.

But before I get into specifics, I want to talk about one of the most essential elements in my program: not eating anything at all.

THE OVERNIGHT FAST

A lot has been written about fasting, a lot of it as good for you as junk food. But the overall principle is the same in all of them: The body needs time to rest from the daily activity of digestion.

Fasting has been the subject of much of my research for more than ten years. I know about the physiology of fasting and about its psychological effects. I've fasted myself numerous times, always keeping journals on my experience. ("Day 2: Today I feel like quitting. I am thinking about all the good food I could be eating . . ." "Morning, Day 5: I feel like a new person. My skin has a glow to it. My eyes are clear. My hunger has not returned yet. It left on Day 3.") Here's what I've found:

When we stop eating, our body goes into autolysis—self-digestion—after the first three days. It begins to break down much of its worn-out, aged tissue, and it eliminates toxins through the bowels and skin. Drinking plenty of water is vital during a fast, and I found that fresh, diluted fruit and vegetable juices, which help with cleansing and nourishment, kept me feeling vital.

Most people fast for the wrong reasons, though, and don't recognize the side effects. Lengthy fasting is *not* the ideal way to lose weight (though you *will* lose weight). And sudden fasts ("Good God! I've gained three pounds in a week. Better not eat anything for three days so I can lose them") sends the body into shock—like showering in ice water after heavy exercise.

The worst results come after the fast ends. The faster, proud of herself and, indeed, having lost a pound or two, immediately begins to binge on the very foods that caused her to panic earlier in the week. "I can eat again," she tells herself, "and if I gain too much weight, I can always go on another fast."

Fasting is not a technique to be used to negate bad eating habits. The fast-famine spiral puts a strain on your entire system. When Cindi came to me, she told me she ate anything she wanted for five days and then fasted for two. "And I don't gain weight," she told me proudly. But her periods were irregular and she suffered from water retention. She had scant sexual interest and she continually felt vaguely depressed, despite a loving boyfriend and a good job.

Her method of eating and fasting had sent her body into metabolic imbalance. In effect, her liver didn't know what was happening to it. The body works optimally when it is on a regular schedule, with few if any surprises. Regularity is the best way to cultivate sexual vitality, too, since the sexual organs are the first to shut down when the body is in shock. So I told Cindi to eliminate the two days of fasting per week and instead to fast for seven nights per week—that is, every night.

As we've seen, the overnight fast, lasting from six P.M. to breakfast (which, remember, is not eaten directly upon arising), gives the body time to clean out without shock treatment. People like to fast—it makes them feel renewed—but if they do it for long periods, they tend to overeat when they stop. With the overnight fast, there is no such tendency. And the therapeutic value is greater. The overnight fast leads to a gradual diminution of appetite rather than the food craving one feels after an extended fast, and it provides enough time for the digestive system to rest for the morning's rejuvenation.

Researchers feel that the overnight fast as described here may contribute to cell renewal to counter oxidative DNA damage caused by free radicals. You'll be rejuvenating your metabolic process and, as a by-product, you'll be training your mind, for if you allow yourself to eat every time your mind tells you that a bite of food would "go good just about now," you'll never train it to be still.

And when you wake up your digestion has been self-cleaning for some twelve hours (do the math: In the course of twenty-one days, you'd be "fasting" for nearly eleven of them!). Break the fast with fresh fruit juice (if you feel you need more of a cleansing because you *did* eat late the night before) or the more nourishing vegetable juice. Or, best of all, my sexual rejuvenator.

QUALITY

You already know that not all food is created equal. Canned beans are inferior to fresh; cartoned orange juice not as nutritious as fresh squeezed. My diet provides recipes based on virgin foods (fresh and chemical-free) as much as possible, but this does not mean you have to be an organic farmer or move your residence from city to countryside.

Good food is found not only in health-food stores (though I forage in them constantly). There are many fresh fruits and vegetables offered in supermarkets today that will enable you to eat healthfully. Indeed, you can eat well even if you're backpacking. I take along prepackaged dried beans, add water to them, cook for six minutes, and have a nutritious dish—even if it's not gourmet cuisine.

And you needn't eat only raw vegetables. Steaming your greens will break down fibers and make the food more digestible, its vitamins more available. You must start out with fresh foods and then work from there.

A few simple additional hints will help you toward sexual vitality.

Grains should be roasted to make them more digestible. Try barley, brown rice, oats, millet, quinoa, rye, buckwheat, and whole wheat.

Fats are required for metabolic function to repair cell membranes. Fish oils, cold-pressed sesame oil, and olive oil are all metabolic enhancers, so eat deep-water ocean fish, tuna, and salmon, in addition to wild game, avocados, almonds, pecans, pine nuts, and pumpkin and sunflower seeds.

Essential proteins can come from meats, fish, or vegetable combinations—and my diet includes them all. In general, avoid beef and be aware that all meats are highly acidifying and many are contaminated with steroids and antibiotics. Stick to wild game, free-range poultry, and seafood. Use animal protein in moderation. From legumes, choose lentils, mung beans, black beans, white beans, navy beans, pinto beans, lima beans, chickpeas, split peas, and tofu, tempeh, and miso.

Dairy products on the whole should be avoided. It is not necessarily the best source for calcium—kale, sesame seeds, kelp, sardines, broccoli, and almonds can supply it. If you need to drink milk, boil it first. Yogurt is good because of its lactobacteria, but it does not aid in promoting sexual vitality.

Vegetables, roots, fruits, and seaweeds perform miracles in the body, but they're insufficient without proteins and fats.

Table salt should be shunned, so use sea salt or tamari instead.

Processed foods should be eliminated.

Refined sugar should be taken in minimum amounts—only sadists would advocate cutting it out entirely.

QUANTITY

While it's better to eat lots of healthy foods than a moderate amount of bad ones, it's still true that the less you eat (within reason), the more weight you'll lose and the more sexually vital you'll feel.

To cut down:

- Chew until solid food becomes liquid—well, *almost* liquid. There's no need to be fanatical.
- Start the meal by eating whole foods. You'll automatically cut down on how much you can consume.
- Don't eat one food first and then another. Start by tasting each one, and then rotate them. When we eat one food first, we never get satisfied.
- Eat your favorite foods first (most kids and many adults save them for last).
- Balance each meal by combining acid foods with alkalizing ones. Start with the alkalizing, such as greens. Then wait ten minutes. The urge to binge will disappear.
- Include herbs and spices. Many times we eat too much due to a need for some flavor. For example, if you just eat plain rice, you'll want some more flavorful food. Spice the rice up with curry or peanut sauce and you'll be satisfied.
- Avoid cold foods and drinks. These lead to overeating. If you drink ice water, you'll want to overeat, so switch to

water at room temperature or warm tea. (Restaurants, I suspect, know this. The more expensive the place, I've found, the more ice you'll get with your water!)

- Kukicha (twig) tea will cut sugar cravings. You can find it in any health-food store.
- When you feel as if you *must* have a bowl of ice cream at night, promise yourself you can have it the next day—at noon.

Of course, there will always be times when you're unable to resist your urges. For those times when you do overeat—you wouldn't be human if you didn't make a pig of yourself sometimes—try the following remedies:

- Don't beat yourself up. Again, you *are* human.
- Drink warm ginger or fennel tea—or kukicha tea, which will counteract the acidity of too much dessert.
- Drink peppermint tea to help digest fats.
- Chew on fennel seeds.
- Fast when it's normally time for your big meal (lunch), confining yourself to vegetable juice or broth.
- To deaden your taste buds (it's only for a little while!), drink dandelion root tea. Its bitters operate on the small intestine, which is most affected by overeating. If you can't stand the tea, try a dried-extract capsule.
- Go back to the vitality diet for an extended period, always remembering how awful you felt when you overate and how unpleasant some of the remedies are.

SUPPLEMENTS

If you follow the vitality diet, you still might need supplements, because many foods are grown in soil depleted of nutrients such as zinc or selenium, or you might be eating too many processed foods, or because you've been overusing the microwave.

Remember, though, that a supplement does not contain or replace the live, organic nutrients found in "real" food. Don't overestimate the power of vitamins.

When deciding on a supplement, opt for a high-potency multiple. I don't recommend isolating vitamins by taking them separately since there's too much chance you'll overdo them, and this can do you more harm than good.

You'll want to make sure your multiple contains the correct amounts, so you'll have to learn to read a label. Get a good vitamin book as an adjunct to this one.

Remember:

- Each of us is biologically and physiologically unique, based on our genes, our experiences, and our lifestyles. A supplement good for one may be ruinous for another.
- Manufacturers are prone to extravagant claims (and use sophisticated marketing techniques) for the thousands of supplements they produce. Don't take them at face value.
- *With the help of a health professional,* determine your needs, establish your objectives, and use the supplements systematically, not just when you feel like it.
- If you do decide on a multiple vitamin, eliminate it for one day each week to clean out any buildup of the fat-soluble vitamins.
- Vitamins and other micronutrients support our biochemical processes and don't create immediate or drastic changes in the body. Give yourself three to four weeks to notice any changes. If none seem to occur, reconsult your doctor.
- *Never self-diagnose!*

Vitamins and minerals that specifically enhance sexual vitality are:

Vitamin A, which is required for healthy epithelial and mucosal cells and has been shown to increase progesterone levels. A deficiency of vitamin A is associated with decreased thyroid levels.

Beta-carotene, which lubricates the vagina, increases progesterone levels, and repairs vaginal tissue.

B-complex, which contributes to the production of sex hormones.

Bioflavonoids, antioxidants, which have a strong estrogenic effect and support the cell membranes.

Vitamin C, an antioxidant, which strengthens cell walls and is required for progesterone secretion.

Vitamin E, which feeds the pituitary and thyroid glands, lubricates the vagina, and supports endocrine glands.

Calcium, which is good for the nervous system and healthy bone function.

Magnesium, which activates enzymes to metabolize amino acids and promotes utilization of other vitamins in maintaining the acid/base balance.

Selenium, which helps protect the body from environmental toxins and is good for the thyroid, which affects libido.

Zinc, which is vital for the proper functioning of the sex glands.

Again, don't mix and match on your own!

HERBS

Different herbs perform different biochemical functions in the body. Some enhance digestion, others eliminate fatigue. Some help clean the liver, others restore the adrenals. Some stimulate blood flow, others shield against toxins. Many maintain or increase sexual vitality. In my recipes, you'll often find herbs included as part of the ingredients.

But herbs can be taken supplementally as well. My only caution is to read the labels if the herb comes packaged, and to buy your herbs from reputable companies—several are listed in the appendix. Herbs are potent—some are even toxic (though none listed in this book). I would caution against mixing too many therapeutic doses of herbs at one time, for they might not complement one another.

If you're just getting familiar with herbs, start with herb teas or tinctures, which are less potent than whole dried extracts, to judge your body's response. If the herb seems to suit you, go on to fresh herbs or dried herbs—but make sure you don't use anything beyond its expiration date. Spices should not be more than six months old. Herbs may have a longer shelf life depending on how they were processed. By the expiration date, the herb will have lost its therapeutic value.

Here are ten spices and herbs used specifically to ignite metabolism and aid the digestive system:

Black peppercorn
Cardamom
Cayenne pepper
Cinnamon
Coriander
Cumin
Fennel
Garlic
Ginger
Turmeric

Spices and herbs like these can be mixed to your liking, but try not to overdo the hot, stimulating ones often used to help digestion. Both black peppercorn and cardamom, for example, aid digestion, but one stimulates the system while the other calms it.

Herbs specifically beneficial to sexual health are the following:

Chaste Tree (VITEX), which nourishes the mucous membrane and promotes progesterone.

Dandelion, which moves the blood, regulates hormones, and acts beneficially on breasts, uterus, and ovaries.

Don quai, often called the "female ginseng," which is considered a rejuvenating female tonic and hormone regulator.

Ginger, which balances the eicosanoids, substances responsible for keeping metabolism in balance.

Gotu kola, considered one of the most important rejuvenative herbs in Ayurvedic medicine, which strengthens the adrenals and purifies the blood.

Licorice, which acts as a rejuvenator of the endocrine system.

Milk thistle, which strengthens the liver and protects against environmental toxins.

Oat straw, which nourishes the nervous and endocrine systems. Some claim it is a great "love potion," that after drinking oat straw tea, they feel sexier and more lubricated.

Siberian ginseng, which supports the adrenals and nervous system.

St. John's wort, a mood elevator that can help relieve depression and anxiety.

Turmeric, which regulates hormone function and promotes proper metabolism.

Wild yam, which is an essential source of zinc.

FLOWER ESSENCES

Like herbs, flower essences can rejuvenate and revitalize. More and more they are being added to the diet, not as an additional "food," but as an aid to psychological well-being. I've seen remarkable results both with single essences and combinations (though no more than three to six at a time), but suggest that if you're interested in persuing flower essences further, you consult a professional practitioner. The best book on the subject is *Flower Essence Repertory: A Comprehensive Guide to North American and English Flower Essences for Emotional and Spiritual*

Well-Being, by Patricia Kaminski and Richard Katz, published in 1994 by the Flower Essence Society, P.O. Box 459, Nevada City, California 95959. Among the flower essences I recommend are pink yarrow, particularly effective during menopause; arnica for the recovery of energy after a trauma; evening primrose, which helps to create intimacy; hibiscus, an aid to warmth and responsiveness in female sexuality; lady's slipper, which helps balance the lower chakras; and snapdragon, which helps develop a strong libido.

One recipe I've found particularly helpful for awakening your own sexuality is this:

In 1 oz. of distilled water, add:
2 drops of brandy (a preservative)
2 drops of self-heal flower essence
2 drops of hibiscus flower essence
2 drops of crab apple flower essence

Mix and take 2 to 4 drops under the tongue four times a day. Do not mix with food fifteen minutes before or after. If you're experiencing a lot of trauma in your life, and can't seem to let go sexually, replace the hibiscus with arnica.

ESSENTIAL OILS

"Essential" means oils that are made from the essence of their basic source. They're not meant to be ingested as part of a diet—indeed, if you imbibe them, you might get sick. And they're not to be used full strength; they must be diluted. But I include them here because they *complement* diet so well when it comes to sexual vitality. I use oils all the time in my bath or when getting or giving a massage. They smell wonderful, relieve stress, relax the body, and quiet the mind—if you've eaten well, they'll even enhance your sexual enjoyment. For example:

Basil, an aromatic nerve tonic, is used to reduce mental fatigue due to stress.

Chamomile relaxes the body by calming the nerves.

Jasmine elevates mood and induces euphoria. It's commonly used as an aphrodisiac.

Lavender reduces stress and relieves headaches.

Neroli, among the finest flower essences, makes a luxurious and relaxing bath or massage oil.

Rose stimulates sexual responsiveness and feelings of sexuality.

Rosemary clears the mind.

Sandlewood relaxes and calms mind and body.

Ylang-ylang, called "the flower of flowers," is commonly used as an aphrodisiac and is one of the most emotionally evocative essential oils.

Experiment with them. What will smell good to one person may turn off another. What stimulates you may be meaningless to your partner. The experimentation is fun. And the results, in case after case, miraculous.

THE VITALITY DIET AND SEX

I've said it before: A dormant sex drive is often the result of an unhealthy body. That's why exercise, breathing, and diet are so important, and why my program will kindle or rekindle your sex life.

Here's how my diet plan relates specifically to sex:

1. Sexual essence requires protein and minerals. My diet includes protein from a number of lean sources and an abundance of minerals from fresh fruits and vegetables.

2. Good sexual performance requires stamina. My diet provides whole grains to balance blood-glucose levels, thus enhancing endurance.

3. Sexual function is controlled by hormones secreted by the endocrine glands. My diet guarantees them proper nutrition.

4. The pituitary gland has both direct and indirect effects on sexual and reproductive functions. Any pituitary deficiency causes underdeveloped sex organs, impotence (in men), and early menopause. My diet recommends foods and vitamin supplements (the B-complex vitamins, vitamin E, zinc, niacin, and so on) specifically geared to the care and feeding of this essential gland.

5. We've seen that the adrenal glands are the seat of sexual vitality. These glands, too, need vitamin-rich foods and supplements. Moreover, I've made sure that my diet avoids adrenal-depleting foods, such as refined sugar and white-flour products.

6. The thyroid gland is correlated with sexual desire and sexual strength. Iodine and several vitamins are essential for the production of its hormones. That's why my diet includes seafood and sea vegetables.

7. The B vitamins, folic acid, niacin, vitamin E, and zinc are essential for the ovaries' production of estrogen and progesterone. My diet will supply them.

8. The sex hormones are made from cholesterol, which is made endogenously and not needed in the diet. Cholesterol-containing foods can be eaten as long as the body has sufficient nutrients to metabolize it. My diet will do this.

9. Sexual desire and performance can be adversely affected by many things, including drugs, alcohol, caffeine, and many common medicines. The vitality diet will rebuild your system—but only if you quit using the substances that sapped your vitality in the first place.

If you follow my diet, you will feel better, look healthier, *be* healthier, and have more energy in your daily life. You'll see its greatest effects, though, in your sexuality.

And your sexuality will be dramatically enhanced if you exercise—particularly your sexual center—and if you learn to breathe properly.

Chapter 10

*B*REATHING FOR
SEXUAL ENERGY

If you master your breath, you master your health—it's as simple as that. Breathing connects all systems in our bodies, by way
of the parasympathetic and sympathetic branches of our nervous system. Nothing happens in our bodies without breath.
The heart can't pump, the brain can't function, hormones can't
flow, and so on. Breathe incorrectly and you will be harming all
systems of the body. Breathe correctly and you are far along on
the road to vitality.

Look at any child from one to five, and you'll see that she
breathes from her diaphragm, the muscle that separates the
upper body from the lower. It's the natural way to breathe, yet
as we grow older and are subjected to anxiety, stress, and fear,
our breathing shifts to the chest, creating unnecessary arousal
and sympathetic activity—physiologists call this a sympathetic
(flight-or-fight) response.

The purpose of this chapter is to teach you a more natural
way to breathe, a way that maximizes respiratory efficiency and
creates balance in the autonomic nervous system. It's the way
you should breathe when you relax and, say, listen to music—
and the way you should breathe if you want to prolong sexual
pleasure. It is called diaphragmatic breathing.

I developed the Metabolic Breathing Training System® for the purpose of rejuvenating the sexual organs and activating metabolism. It begins with diaphragmatic breathing, a smooth, unbroken expansion of the lungs that begins at the bottom, not at the top. This method of breathing cuts down on the number of breaths per minute, saves work on the heart, and boosts blood circulation, sending blood coursing strongly throughout the system. When the diaphragm is fully expanded, the intercostal muscles open the rib cage and fill the mid-lungs with air. In the metabolic breathing method, the breather maintains the full expansion of the rib cage, as in diaphragmatic breathing. The difference lies in the exhalation. Instead of being passive, it is an active exhalation. During exhalation the breather uses a slight abdominal lift, its purpose being to "ignite the metabolic fire." Systematically combining diaphragmatic breathing with the active abdominal lift, the breather will tone her female organs, promote vitality, and bring a lustrous glow to her face. It is truly a beauty potion.

The exercises that follow are taken from both ancient and modern sources. They have been modified in some cases to make them easier for the average person (you and me), but they'll do the job: They'll revitalize you.

We begin with the nostrils. As noted, most people are oblivious to which nostril is dominant at any given time. If you came to me feeling lethargic and uninterested in sex, my first question would be "Which nostril feels more air flow?" If you didn't know, my next question would be "How can you expect to change your present physical state?" Nostril breathing should be deep, slow, constant, smooth, natural, regular, silent, and gentle—with an inhalation/exhalation ratio of 1:1.

I've already discussed the sexual benefits of alternate-nostril breathing; now is the time to explain why and show you how.

Nasal breathing is much preferred to mouth breathing for a variety of reasons. The inner nose performs nearly thirty functions, among them the filtering, warming, and moisturizing of incoming air, and it is responsible for the ability to smell, which affects the limbic system, the seat of emotion.

ALTERNATE-NOSTRIL BREATHING EXERCISE

Purpose

To alternate the flow of air between right and left nostrils, thus balancing the energy channels associated with the right and left nostril and right and left hemispheres of the brain. Once mastered, an excellent means for focusing the mind during sexual activity.

Technique

1. Sit in a chair, with head, neck, and trunk aligned.
2. Bring your right hand to the nose, folding the pinky, index finger, and middle finger so that the right thumb can be used to close the right nostril and the ring finger can be used to close the left nostril.
3. Close the passive nostril and exhale completely through the active nostril.
4. At the end of the exhalation, close the active nostril and slowly inhale through the passive nostril. Inhalation and exhalation should be of equal duration.
5. Repeat the cycle of exhalation with the active nostril and inhalation with the passive nostril three times.
6. At the end of the third inhalation with the passive nostril, exhale completely through the *same* nostril, keeping the active nostril closed with the finger or thumb.
7. At the end of the exhalation, close the passive nostril and inhale through the active nostril.
8. Exhale through the passive nostril and inhale through the active nostril three times.
9. Place your hands on your knees and exhale and inhale through both nostrils evenly for three complete breaths.

This completes one cycle of alternate-nostril breathing. You should be completely aware of the process. At the beginning, repeat several times during the day until it becomes natural.

DIAPHRAGMATIC BREATHING

The human body was designed for diaphragmatic breathing, but many of us keep our diaphragms frozen. This limits sensitivity and awareness and increases stress. Breathe through your chest when you're making love, and I guarantee you that the sex will not be as pleasurable as when you breathe from the diaphragm.

Diaphragmatic breathing is both energizing and relaxing. The breathing apparatus includes the trachea, which allows air to pass into the lungs; the lungs, which are the organs where gas exchange takes place; the diaphragm, which lengthens and shortens the chest cavity; and the rib cage, which creates the structure and protection of the breathing apparatus.

The diaphragm is the resilient, flexible muscular membrane that separates the chest cavity from the abdominal cavity. When the lungs expand, they push the diaphragm downward; when the lungs contract, they pull it toward the chest cavity. When the diaphragm is used for breathing, the chest remains motionless, but other parts of the torso, and particularly the abdomen, move slightly. As you refine and perfect your breathing, this motion becomes increasingly subtle.

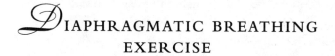

$\mathcal{D}$IAPHRAGMATIC BREATHING
EXERCISE

Purpose

To teach you how to breathe with the abdomen and isolate the diaphragm. This exercise is the foundation for all the exercises that follow.

Technique

1. Begin by lying on your back with your knees bent and your feet flat on the floor. Place a one- to three-pound book on your abdomen and observe your breath. (You may use a rock if you're outdoors and don't have a book with you.)
2. On inhalation, allow your abdomen to expand and the book to rise. Exhale and watch the book lower.
3. Repeat this exercise in fifteen-minute sessions until it becomes natural, when you will no longer need the book.

METABOLIC BREATHING

Metabolic breathing was developed from ancient yoga breathing practices, for the yoga masters recognized early that by controlling their breath, they would gain access to controlling their health and longevity. Metabolic breathing modifies and combines some of these practices, in particular abdominal breathing, diaphragmatic breathing, and *agni sara*. (As you'll see, I've added a slight lift, specifically meant to ignite the metabolic fire.) *Agni sara* literally means "energizing the solar system," but here the "solar system" refers to the interconnection of the psychological and physiological processes that control our digestion and influence our reproductive, circulatory, and nervous systems. It focuses on the lower abdomen, extending two to three inches below the navel, the locus of the second and third chakras. If you combine this breathing method with your exercise, and practice it at other times during the day, you will tone your sex organs and bring the glow to your face that indicates a steadily burning metabolic fire.

Metabolic breathing is designed to expel stale residual air and toxins from the deepest recesses of the lungs, in order to clear and open all passages in the throat and head (it is especially valuable for smokers and city dwellers). The concommitant rise in oxygen levels revitalizes the blood, and in its journey throughout the body especially stimulates the metabolism. Extra oxygen infusions are calming to the nervous system, stimulating to the digestion, and beneficial to the adrenal glands. Metabolic breathing is not something you should do all day, but it is a marvelous aid to sexual pleasure, and it will actually help the digestive process after a too-large meal.

*M*ETABOLIC BREATHING

Purpose

To invigorate the metabolism by providing increased circulation and vitality to the sexual organs and digestive system.

Technique

1. Follow the procedure for diaphragmatic breathing.
2. On exhalation, provide an extra lift with the lower abdominal muscles, as if you were stopping your urine from flowing.
3. Breathe evenly through both nostrils with no jerks or pauses.
4. When combined with exercise, adjust each movement to the breathing to correspond to one inhalation and one exhalation.

*B*ELLOWS EXERCISE

Purpose

To expel toxins from the body and rejuvenate the energy system.

Technique

Sitting with head, neck, and trunk in a straight line, place your tongue against your palate and keep it there throughout the exercise.

Start by forcefully expelling all air from the lungs through the nostrils, combined with a strong contraction of the abdominal wall. Immediately afterward, let the lungs fill without force. Repeat this exercise for fifteen to thirty seconds. End with a complete inhalation and exhalation. Do not practice while exercising.

COMPLETE BREATH EXERCISE

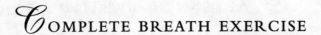

Purpose

To expand the capacity of the lungs and energize the body and mind.

Technique

Choose a well-ventilated area. Either standing or lying down, begin inhaling from the abdomen, then the middle area, then the upper chest. As you inhale, simultaneously raise your hands over your head till your palms are touching. Repeat three times.

Note: Metabolic breathing shifts all your attention to your breath. It means attending to your breath as it enters the nostrils, expands the abdominal region, and flows out the nasal passages, thus keeping other distractions at bay. As a result, you bring the autonomic nervous system into a balanced, more relaxed mode while invigorating the organ systems in your body. Ultimately, it becomes the connection between body and mind.

Chapter 11

EXERCISES THAT ENERGIZE

Beth came for an appointment. She felt she was carrying excess weight around her abdomen, hips, and thighs, and she wanted to put together a workout specifically to meet her female needs. Her diet was reasonable, I found, though we made some adjustments. When I asked her about sexual activity, she claimed she hadn't had sex in a year. She slouched and breathed from her chest, obvious reflections of the condition of her mind.

As I had requested when she first called, she was wearing sweatclothes. "Lie down on the mat," I said.

She did.

"I'm going to start you on some leg exercises."

When I demonstrated my V exercises, I was not surprised that her legs remained closed.

"With your legs together, lift your knees to your chest."

She couldn't do it.

I supported her legs and gradually worked on rotating them out and open. After several sessions, Beth learned to both open her legs and raise them. Soon she reported that she did not feel the excess weight. Eventually, too, she and her lover began making love again.

The purpose of my exercise program is to activate the second and third chakras, and this is what Beth accomplished. If you follow the exercises prescribed here (along with good diet and breathing—as I keep saying, the three are inextricably intertwined), you will feel your body open like a flower and experience your full feminine nature. There are exercises of the neck, chest, and shoulders that will release stress and tension, but my aim here is strictly sexual. When we imprison our sexuality, we imprison ourselves. When we let our sexuality free, we find our whole selves; we find freedom.

Mind you, I have nothing against aerobics *if they're done skillfully,* but most of us do them poorly. (I shudder at the sight of bent-over women huffing and puffing on a StairMaster. They're putting stress on the body as opposed to building it.) I recommend t'ai chi and yoga, not so much for their physical effects but because they help maintain a balance between mind and body. (Be sure your teacher is aware of the importance of the breath.) And I endorse lifting weights because most women have not developed their upper-body strength to the maximum potential, which causes them to slouch when they walk, making it difficult to open the heart center. But all these are not as important for sexual vitality as the exercises prescribed here.

Awareness is the first step in changing any aspect of yourself, and exercise is a great way to become aware of your body. But it is essential to remember that exercise and breathing (just like sex and breathing) are inextricably intertwined, and actually you should be sure to have read the chapter on breath before starting on the exercises I recommend.

My program begins with posture. You must learn to "let your genitals do the walking"—that is, stand straight and walk with your pelvis open along with the rest of your body. Unless you can do this, your sexual vitality will be limited and the exercises won't have their full effect. When your spinal column is not straight and steady, both psychological and physiological issues arise. When you're depressed, for example, you tend to let your head droop. This posture will in turn create a feedback loop that will keep you in a depressed state. Unless you extend the spine and hold your head, neck, and trunk straight, your breathing will be affected, and this also will affect your mood. A balanced body provides a foundation for balance on every level of our being, including energy, mind, and spirit.

Before starting the exercises, try "body scanning." Later in the chapter, I'll teach you the optimum method, but for now stop reading for a moment and close your eyes. You should be able to detect different sensations throughout your body. Does the left side of your face feel the same as the right side? Do your shoulders feel heavy or light? When you stand, do both feet put equal pressure on the floor or are you depending more on one than the other? The more we become aware of how our bodies *feel,* the easier it will be to balance them through exercise.

Finally, there are the exercises themselves. They are designed to develop muscles without stiffness so that energy runs free, to revitalize organs such as the liver, kidneys, and lungs, as well as the reproductive organs. One aim is to increase respiration, much as aerobic exercise does. Yoga techniques are employed that incorporate both tension and relaxation.

YOUR EXERCISE SELF-EVALUATION

Before beginning any exercise program, you must ask yourself two questions: "What is my goal?" and "How is my health?" The exercises here assume your health is good, and that you want to stimulate your metabolism so that you can maintain or promote sexual vitality and add longevity to it.

As you exercise, evaluate your appetite, both for food and for sex, and record your recovery time. Do you become ravenous for food within two hours of exercising? If so, you're probably exercising too much. (It's easy to *gain* weight through exercising. All it takes is the thought that "I've burned off five hundred calories. I deserve a snack.") Does your desire for sex decrease after a week of hard workouts? Again, you're probably exercising too much. In fact, exercise can be a sex substitute. Too much will deplete your sexual fluids, and overexercising, particularly in concert with overeating, will cause you to lose the softness and grace that comes with being sexually radiant. Hardness sets in. Passion is driven out. If you find yourself preferring to exercise rather than go out on a date, you're in trouble.

Evaluate your desire for further exercise. If you feel enthusiastic about the next workout, good! If, on the other hand, you drag yourself to the exercise room, feeling fatigued and disheartened, take a day off. Or take two. (But don't take three.) If you haven't been exercising regularly, you may feel uncomfortable at first, but even if there's a little muscle soreness, you can still feel good. Determine for yourself the difference between being mildly uncomfortable and needing a rest or recovery period.

EXERCISE REGULARITY AND CONSISTENCY

Some people are more energetic in the morning, others at night. If possible, exercise when you feel most energetic (before work or after, before breakfast or after dinner), but *be consistent*. Discipline means shaping desired behavior. Find what works for you, not for your friends. It's fun to exercise in tandem with a friend, but choose one with a similar energy pattern. You'll both benefit.

In general, exercising in the morning is usually better for those people just starting out or those who have trouble sticking to a program. As noted, it saves you the problem of having the time to think about not doing it, and it fends off excuses like "I've had a tough day at the office" or "I walked a lot anyway." As we've seen, one drawback to morning exercise is that you're likely to feel slightly more hungry during the day. Resist the impulse to add to your lunch and avoid the mid-morning snack.

Afternoons are probably the hardest time to exercise, since this is when our blood sugar is low and we want a quick pick-me-up rather than an hour of working out. But it may deter the binge eating that often occurs in the late afternoon.

Exercising in the evening will relax you, particularly if you do it after dinner and don't eat afterward. It'll probably give you the greatest metabolic boost, too, resulting in greater weight loss if this is your goal.

DURATION AND FREQUENCY

Pick your time of day, *and stick to it for twenty-one days.* That's how long the body takes to adapt to exercise and to change. After the three weeks are over, make an evaluation. If you're seeing results, continue at the same pace for the next fourteen days, at which time you might want to move on to a more difficult level.

Research shows that people who exercise four or five days a week lose weight three times faster than those who exercise two times a week. Translating this to your metabolism, you'll find that the same schedule holds true. There is no permanent change without regular exercise, but remember that moderate, sustained exercise is far better for sexual vitality than vigorous exertion.

SUPPLEMENTARY EXERCISING

The use of weights and other devices—extra resistance of any kind during a workout—will increase muscle endurance and strength. It may also increase the heart rate, depending on the speed, intensity, and duration of the activity with which you're employing resistance. There's no question that it can help develop the muscle, tendon, and ligament strength needed to balance the body. I don't emphasize resistance training in my program—really, you should build up to it over time—but I recognize its importance and if you think you're up to it, go for it.

As for aerobics, my program does include a workout that if performed at the highest level will provide aerobic conditioning. But usually it's best just to add activities such as cycling, fast walking, jogging, or swimming to your weekly routine.

My program includes flexibility training that goes beyond the simple stretching that all of us should do before any extended exercise. Combined with metabolic breathing, it will allow you to control any aspect of your physical functioning, including before, during, and after sex.

EXERCISE GUIDELINES

- Follow the breathing instructions in Chapter 10 as you exercise.
- As noted, choose the best time of day to do the exercises consistently and systematically. Be flexible with the time at the beginning to see what suits you best.
- Do your exercising on an empty stomach. If that's too difficult, drink a cup of tea or diluted fruit juice before you start. Optimally, wait an hour after a light meal and two to three hours after a heavy meal before you start. Remember, it's hard to breathe properly if your digestive system is still working on the last meal.
- Find a clean, well-ventilated room where you can be comfortable. Make sure there are no distractions. Turn off the phone and prohibit child (or spousal) interference. As I've said, it's okay to exercise with a friend, but she must be as

dedicated as you. If you want music, fine. But make sure it doesn't distract you from your breath awareness.

- Create a habit that will let you continue beyond the first days or weeks. If you feel exhilarated by the exercises, you know you're doing something right. Begin by thinking of these exercises as a way of observing yourself. One aim is to change the imbalances in your body (discovered through body scanning), but this takes time.

- Do not be discouraged by the lack of a sudden "hit" or epiphany. The benefits of exercise come in time, and the time will come faster if you're having fun.

- My exercises are intended for women in good health. If you have a condition that warrants medical attention, get your doctor's okay before starting the program. Pregnant and postpartum women should also check with their doctor first. And the metabolic breathing technique is not to be used if you're pregnant or menstruating.

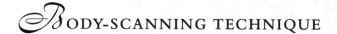ODY-SCANNING TECHNIQUE

Purpose

To be aware of where tension resides in your body so you can release it. Once you know where the problems lie, you'll be able to form your own program of exercises.

Technique

Stand. Put your left heel into the instep of your right foot, then slide the left heel away from the right foot so that your heels are aligned (your feet will be approximately twelve inches apart) and your weight is balanced evenly over your hips. Close your eyes and begin scanning by "observing" the lightness or heaviness you feel in various parts of your body. Begin with the neck, followed by the upper back. Continue to the shoulders, hips, pelvis, thighs, knees, calves, and feet.

Remain in the standing position for three minutes after you've completed the scan, paying attention to your thought processes. When a thought comes to your attention, notice the effect it has on your body. If you feel your shoulders tighten, say, or your thighs grow tense, you'll know which exercises to try.

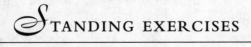

$\mathcal{S}$TANDING EXERCISES

Purpose

To build body heat, strength, and endurance. The exercises are designed to increase the flexibility of the legs and upper body while toning the front and back of the thighs and increasing upper-body definition. The bending adds to the flexibility of the spine and promotes vitality. Many women carry weight on their hips and thighs, making them feel less sexually vital. The standing exercises will aid in increasing lean muscle tissue and promoting fat loss.

Overall Technique

Keep the spine as straight as possible. Maintain straight posture rather than letting yourself slump. Weight should be evenly distributed on your feet.

$\mathscr{C}$ELESTIAL BREATH

Purpose

Balancing the mind-body connection.

Technique

Feet should be shoulder-distance apart. Stand with knees bent, as if you are about to sit on a raised stool. Spine must be kept straight with hands placed palms down on your lower abdomen.

Exhale totally and begin using metabolic breathing, inhaling through the nose. As you inhale, slowly raise your hands, palms up, out to your sides and inscribe as wide a circle with them as possible. At the same time, slowly straighten your knees so you are standing upright.

Bring your palms together when your hands are overhead, making sure your lungs are full at the same time. Stretch from your ankles to the top of your head. Hold the stretch for three breaths and then release. Repeat the exercise three times.

Beginner level.

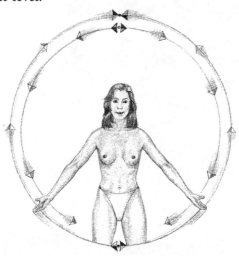

$\mathcal{H}$IP CIRCLES

Purpose

To open and energize the second chakra.

Technique

Feet should be shoulder-distance apart. Stand with knees bent, as if you are about to sit on a raised stool. Keep spine straight. Place hands on hips. Begin by rotating to the right and then to the left, leading with your pelvis as though you are dancing. Increase the amount of the turn each time. Repeat until you have reached the maximum turn.

Beginner level.

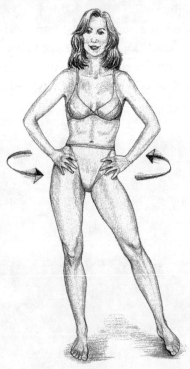

$\mathcal{W}$INDMILLS

Purpose

To release tension in the body and allow energy to move upward.

Technique

Feet should be shoulder-distance apart. Stand with knees bent, as if you are about to sit on a raised stool. Keep spine and pelvis straight. Begin swinging your arms from side to side across your body, allowing your head to turn with your body, increasing the length of swing with each repetition. As you swing, let your arms gently hit your body. Repeat several times.

Beginner level.

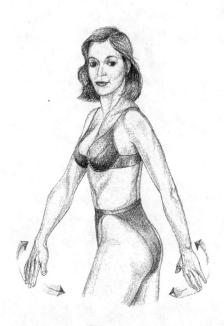

$\mathscr{S}$TANDING CAT

Purpose

To create a flexible spine and release tension in the neck and shoulders.

Technique

Stand with feet shoulder-distance apart. With knees slightly bent, bend over and bring your hands down to your knees. With an exhalation, bring your chin into your chest as you round your back. On inhalation, bring your chin away from your chest and slowly arch your back. Repeat, letting the right shoulder drop as you turn to look over your left shoulder. Repeat, letting the left shoulder drop as you look over your right shoulder. Hold the positions as long as they seem comfortable. With each repeat, extend the length of stretch.

Beginner level.

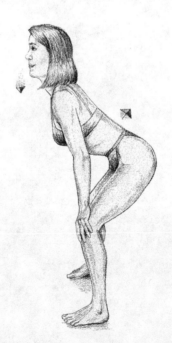

THE TURTLE

Purpose

To energize the legs and release lower-body tension.

Technique

Stand with your legs spread apart as much as possible without losing balance. With an exhalation, bend over with your knees slightly bent, trying to touch your palms to the floor. (Beginners should put palms on thighs.) Look up, maintaining a flat back—imagine pushing your tailbone to the ceiling. On inhalation, straighten your knees and maintain palms on the floor. Repeat two or three times.

Beginner through advanced level.

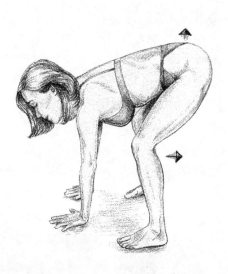

THE SQUAT

Purpose

To strengthen the legs and butt.

Technique

Stand with your feet spread twelve inches more than shoulder-width apart, toes out 10 to 25 degrees. Inhale as you bend your knees, slowly sinking down as if about to sit on a stool. Keep your weight on your heels, thighs parallel to the floor, and knees over your ankles, not your toes. Exhale and rise to a standing position. As you come up, draw the PC muscle upward, as if you were sucking in energy from the earth. Then release.

Beginner level. When you are more advanced, you may hold weights in your hands, which are resting on your thighs.

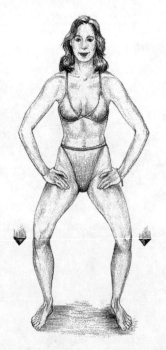

$\mathcal{T}$HE LUNGE

Purpose

To stretch and tone the pelvic region by enhancing the mobility of hip and groin muscles.

Technique

Stand with feet shoulder-distance apart, arms down at your sides. Step forward with the left foot, maintaining balance but enough to feel a stretch. Keep weight on the heel of the left foot to keep pressure off the knee. On an inhalation, slowly lower your body until the left thigh is parallel to the floor. Then exhale and come up slowly. Repeat, switching sides each time.

Beginner level. Intermediates may add hand-held weights, advancing the weights and adding a front kick as you come up.

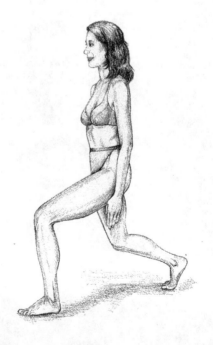

$\mathcal{W}$OOD CHOPPER

Purpose

Lessens fatigue in the upper back and opens the fourth chakra.

Technique

Stand with feet shoulder-distance apart. Interlock fingers behind your back. On an exhalation, with knees slightly bent, bend over and bring your arms forward, keeping your fingers interlocked. As you round your back, put your chin on your chest. On an inhalation, bring your chin away from your chest and arch your back, keeping your arms behind you. Come to an upright position, unlocking your fingers and bringing your arms to your sides. Repeat four to six times.

Beginner through advanced level.

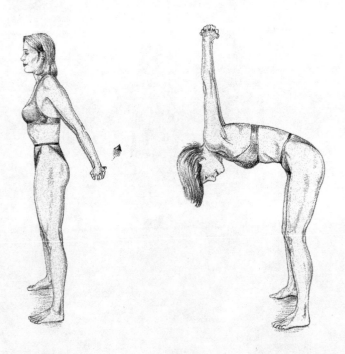

$\mathcal{P}$IKE POSITION

Purpose

To lessen fatigue and restore lost energy.

Technique

Lie facedown, feet shoulder-distance apart, balls of feet on the floor. Keep your arms by your sides, palms flat on the floor. Inhale, arching your back without pressure from your arms, moving your chin away from your chest. Straighten your arms and expand your chest. Exhale as you lower your chin to your chest, and begin to raise your buttocks into the air, extending the stretch down the back of your legs and pressing the heels of your feet against the floor. Repeat several times.

Beginner through advanced level. As you get stronger, only your feet and hands will touch the floor.

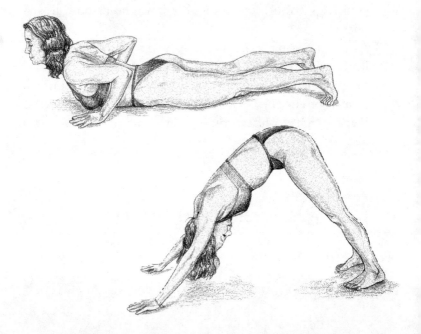

ℒEG LIFTS

Purpose

To specifically increase your sexual vitality. Added benefits include toning the legs and stimulating the reproductive organs.

Overall Technique

All leg exercises will follow the same basic steps:

1. Lie on your back. Before beginning leg exercises, support your back by resting on your elbows. Absolute beginners can lie with head down and hands wedged under the buttocks. If you feel discomfort in your neck or lower back, adjust your position until there is no discomfort.
2. Begin each exercise by tucking your chin into your chest and inhaling as you lift your leg(s). Inhale each time you lift your leg(s). You may lift one leg at a time or both legs at once.
3. As you lift each leg, be sure to extend it from your body, as if you were trying to elongate the muscles.
4. While exhaling, lower the leg(s) and begin to lift your chin from your chest.
5. Repeat eight to fifteen times, depending on your strength and endurance.

𝒮INGLE STRAIGHT LIFTS

Follow Steps 1 to 5, starting with the left leg then going on to the right.

Beginner level.

$\mathscr{D}$OUBLE LIFTS

Follow Steps 1 to 5, raising both legs simultaneously. If you have discomfort in your lower back while lifting both legs, bend your knees until your abdominals get stronger.

Intermediate/advanced level.

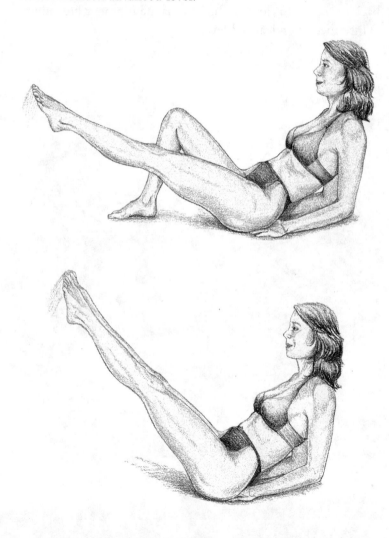

ℰNERGY PUMP

Follow Step 1. Then tuck your knees into your chest. Press the left heel away from your body while the right leg stays close to your chest. Alternate legs. (It's like riding a bicycle.) As you get more adept, you can lower your legs closer to the floor. Keep back straight. Go slow enough to maintain proper breathing.

Intermediate/advanced level.

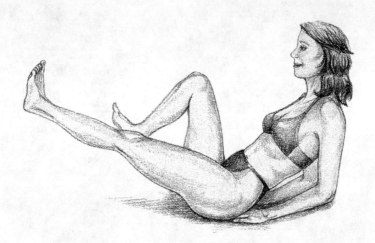

$\mathscr{H}$IP RELEASER

Sit on the floor with a pillow under your buttocks. Spread your legs apart, making a **V**. Place your hands in front of you on the floor to support your upper body. Begin making circles with your body in a clockwise direction. Repeat, going counter-clockwise.

Beginner level.

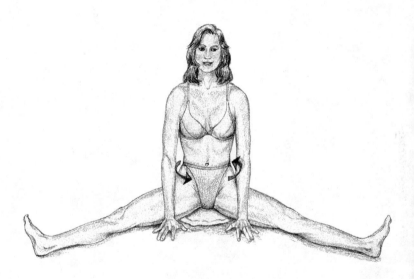

ℋIP RELEASER II

Follow Step 1. On inhalation, spread your legs apart, making a
V. Close on exhalation.
  Intermediate level.

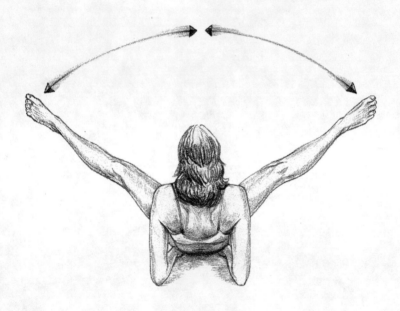

$\mathscr{A}$ROUND THE WORLD

Follow Step 1. Extend both legs to the ceiling, keeping back flat on the floor. On inhalation, open your legs and begin circling them toward the outside. Circle them five times, then rest. Reverse, making five inward circles. The larger the circles, the more difficult the exercise. To start, repeat three times.

Advanced level.

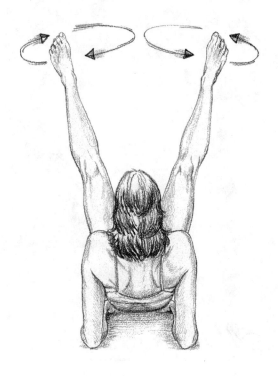

METABOLIC MASTER

From a supine position, rise and balance on your buttocks (hands underneath for balance if need be); bring your knees to your chest, toes pointed. Keep your head and neck tucked. Inhale, opening your body like a flower, arms extended over your head, legs extended out.

Intermediate level.

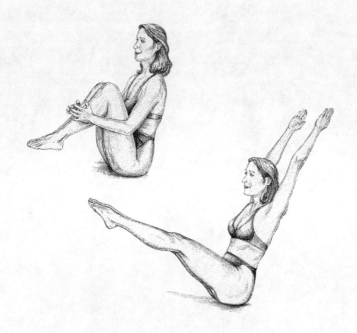

METABOLIC MASTER II

Lie flat on your back, arms overhead, legs extended, feet together. Inhale, raising your lower and upper body until you roll onto your hips. Try to make a ninety-degree angle. Keep back straight. Hold for three seconds, then exhale and lower your body.

Advanced level.

ᴄHE TWIST

Purpose

To increase flexibility of the spine and relieve tension. You'll also be help-ing your metabolism by increasing blood flow to the digestive system.

Technique

Lie on your back and draw your knees to your chest. Extend both arms out to the side. Keeping your shoulders on the floor, rotate knees to one side as you exhale. Repeat to the other side. Do this a minimum of three or four times.

Beginner level.

(In a variation called the Pretzel Twist, the legs are inter-twined. Let them fall to one side, then the other. This opens the pelvis. Intermediate level.)

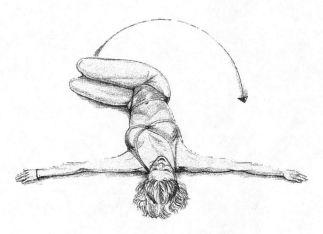

$\mathcal{I}$NVERTED PELVIC LIFTS

Purpose

To tone the endocrine system.

$\mathcal{R}$OCKING

Technique

From a supine position, bring your knees to your chest. Raise your head. Begin a rocking motion forward and back, massaging your spine. As you become more flexible, you can begin to straighten your legs.

Beginner level.

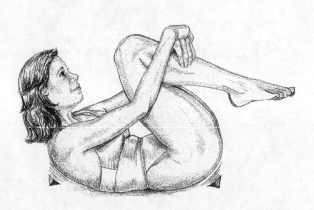

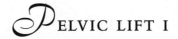ELVIC LIFT I

Technique

Lie on your back and bend your knees, keeping your feet flat on the floor and your hands extended down at your sides. On inhalation, slowly roll up one vertebrae at a time, bringing the pelvis upward toward the ceiling, keeping shoulders and head flat on the floor, and not using the arms for leverage. Exhale, slowly bringing your body down to the starting position. Repeat five times in unison with the breath.

Beginner level.

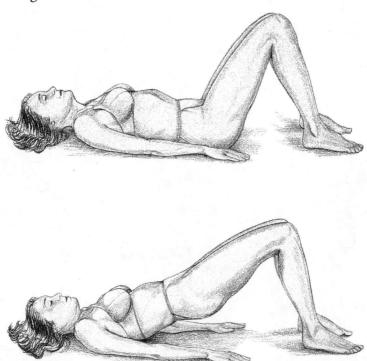

℘ELVIC LIFT II

Technique

Sit on the floor with your knees bent, legs shoulder-width apart, feet flat on the floor, and hands palm down with fingers facing forward. Exhale and tuck chin to chest. Slowly inhale, untucking your chin as you slowly lift your body and extend your pelvis toward the ceiling. Hold. Repeat five times.

Intermediate to advanced level.

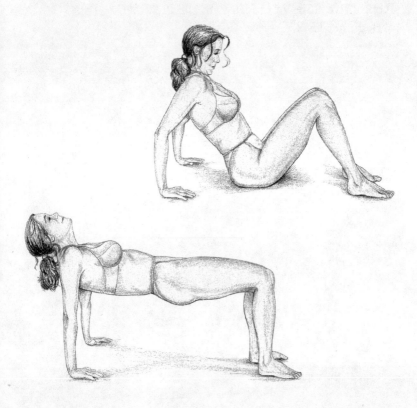

Diet, breathing, exercise. Here's how they work together in my twenty-one-day program.

$\mathscr{C}$HE START-UP 21-DAY PLAN

NOTES

- Desserts are not included in the menus but are optional at lunch.
- An asterisk denotes that the recipe is included herein (see pages 195–223).
- Breathing and exercise, which are to be done every day, are described at the end of the plan.
- Preferably, all food should be eaten before seven P.M.
- Breakfast should be eaten before eight A.M.
- Consult your physician before conducting an overnight fast or eliminating dairy products entirely from your diet.

MENUS

Day 1

UPON ARISING
Sexual Rejuvenator*

BREAKFAST
Metabolic Cleanser*
Flaxseed Cereal with Soy Milk* (optional)

LUNCH
Baked Falafel*
Steamed string beans
Whole-grain bread with topping
Beverage
Dessert (optional)

DINNER
Miso soup
Gingered fish
Mixed Steamed Greens*
Warm beverage

Day 2

UPON ARISING
Sexual Rejuvenator*

BREAKFAST
Hormone Balancer*
Rice Cereal with Soy Milk* (optional)

LUNCH
Grilled chicken sandwich
Wild-Rice Salad*
Beverage
Dessert (Optional)

DINNER
Vegetarian burger
Roasted Rice*

Broccoli with olive oil and lemon
Warm beverage

Day 3

UPON ARISING
Sexual Rejuvenator*

BREAKFAST
Fresh Fruit Plate with Granola Topping*
Toasted Oats* (optional)

LUNCH
Pizza Linguine Style*
Energy Salad with Olive Oil/Garlic or Classic Vinaigrette
    Dressing*
Beverage
Dessert (optional)

DINNER
Black-bean soup
Steamed garlic broccoli
Warm beverage

Day 4

UPON ARISING
Sexual Rejuvenator*

BREAKFAST
Vitality Promoter*
Blueberry bran muffin (optional)

LUNCH
Phytoestrogen Delight*

Whole-grain toasted bread
Fresh fruit
Beverage
Dessert (optional)

DINNER
Broiled salmon with lemon
Steamed rice
Energy Salad*
Warm beverage

Day 5

UPON ARISING
Sexual Rejuvenator*

BREAKFAST
Fresh grapefruit juice
Muesli cereal with soy milk (optional)

LUNCH
Pasta Pesto*
Whole-grain muffin with fruit spread
Beverage
Dessert (optional)

DINNER
Mineral Mountain*
Stuffed Zucchini*
Green salad with olive-oil vinaigrette
Warm beverage

Day 6

UPON ARISING
Sexual Rejuvenator*

BREAKFAST
Banana Soy Shake*
Sweet Fruit Salad* (optional)

LUNCH
Vegetable Bean Pie*
Sprouted Rye Bread with Hummus Spread*
Beverage
Dessert (optional)

DINNER
Thyroid Balancer (kelp soup)*
Baked turkey breast
Sautéed vegetables
Baked potato
Warm beverage

Day 7

UPON ARISING
Sexual Rejuvenator*

BREAKFAST
Mixed berries
Toasted Oatmeal with Soy Milk and Raisins* (optional)

LUNCH
Fatigue Eliminator*
Lentil Soup*
Energy Salad*
Beverage
Dessert (optional)

DINNER
Broiled scallops with lemon
Asparagus with Honey-Lemon Dressing*

Scalloped potatoes with greens
Warm beverage

Day 8

UPON ARISING
Sexual Rejuvenator*

BREAKFAST
Fresh vegetable or fruit juice
Egg-white omelet with peppers and onions (optional)

LUNCH
Stuffed Eggplant*
Steamed collards with olive oil and lemon
Beverage
Dessert (optional)

DINNER
Grilled Shrimp, Mushrooms, and Snow Peas on a Bed of
  Rice*
Green salad
Warm beverage

Day 9

UPON ARISING
Sexual Rejuvenator*

BREAKFAST
Fresh fruit
Dry cereal with berries and soy milk (optional)

LUNCH
Pasta with Tofu and Tomato Pesto Sauce*
Arugula salad with balsamic vinegar

Beverage
Dessert (optional)

DINNER
Poached tilapia
Garlicky Greens*
Fruit sorbet
Warm beverage

Day 10

UPON ARISING
Sexual Rejuvenator*

BREAKFAST
Vitality Promoter*
Toasted oatmeal with soy milk, raisins, and spices (optional)

LUNCH
Tabouleh*
Energy Salad*
Beverage
Dessert (optional)

DINNER
Marinated Tofu*
Steamed greens
Warm beverage

Day 11

UPON ARISING
Sexual Rejuvenator*

BREAKFAST
Grapefruit juice
Whole-grain muffin with apple butter (optional)

LUNCH
Tuna melt
Sea Vegetable Salad*
Beverage
Dessert (optional)

DINNER
Baked turkey breast
Herbed rice
Broccoli spears with lemon
Warm beverage

Day 12

UPON ARISING
Sexual Rejuvenator*

BREAKFAST
Metabolic Cleanser*
Stewed prunes with whole-grain muffin (optional)

LUNCH
Swiss Chard Pizza*
Mixed green salad
Beverage
Dessert (optional)

DINNER
Pepper/Tomato/Basil Salad*
Chickpeas in Hot Tomato Sauce*
Wild-rice salad
Warm beverage

Day 13

UPON ARISING
Sexual Rejuvenator*

BREAKFAST
Fruit Smoothie*
Baked muffin with apple butter (optional)

LUNCH
Lentil Salad in Pita Bread*
Fruit sorbet
Beverage

DINNER
Poached cod with tomato, parsley, and garlic
Sautéed greens
Seasoned rice
Warm beverage

Day 14

UPON ARISING
Sexual Rejuvenator*

BREAKFAST
Vitality Promoter*
Eggless Tofu* with whole-grain bread and almond butter
  (optional)

LUNCH
Vegetable-bean soup
Whole-grain bread
Beverage
Dessert (optional)

DINNER
Ratatouille Over Rice*
Cucumber Salad with Vinaigrette*
Warm beverage

Day 15

UPON ARISING
Sexual Rejuvenator*

BREAKFAST
Fruit Smoothie*
Egg-White Omelet with Mushrooms and Tofu* (optional)

LUNCH
Soup of choice
Spinach salad with whole-grain roll
Beverage
Dessert (optional)

DINNER
Baked fish with fresh herbs
Sautéed Brussels Sprouts*
Warm beverage

Day 16

UPON ARISING
Sexual Rejuvenator*

BREAKFAST
Vegetable-Apple Juice Cocktail*
Zucchini Bread* (optional)

LUNCH
Cold Pasta Salad with Tomato, Basil, and Tofu*
Energy Salad*
Beverage
Dessert (optional)

DINNER
Protein burger
Grilled vegetables
Pineapple wedges

Day 17

UPON ARISING
Sexual Rejuvenator*

BREAKFAST
Fruit or juice
Granola with soy milk (optional)

LUNCH
Traditional chicken salad or Tofu Chicken Salad* on whole-grain bread
Beverage
Dessert (optional)

DINNER
Curried tofu
Stir-fried Greens with Ginger*
Fresh fruit
Warm beverage

Day 18

UPON ARISING
Sexual Rejuvenator*

BREAKFAST
Fresh fruit
Toasted Oatmeal with Soy Milk and Banana* (optional)

LUNCH
Garden Burger*
Endive salad
Beverage
Dessert (optional)

DINNER
Marinated Shrimp and Chicken Kebobs with Grilled
   Vegetables*
Herbed rice
Warm beverage

Day 19

UPON ARISING
Sexual Rejuvenator*

BREAKFAST
Apple juice
Toasted whole-grain bread with apple butter (optional)

LUNCH
Whole-grain sandwich with onion and tomato
Light Vegetable Broth*
Beverage
Dessert (optional)

DINNER
Mineral Mountain*
Tempeh Vegetable Stir-fry*
Warm beverage

Day 20

UPON ARISING
Sexual Rejuvenator*

BREAKFAST
Vitality Promoter*
Dry cereal with berries

LUNCH
Couscous Salad*
Mixed Steamed Greens*
Beverage
Dessert (optional)

DINNER
Rosemary chicken
Rice pilaf
Green salad
Warm beverage

Day 21

UPON ARISING
Sexual Rejuvenator*

BREAKFAST
Hormone Balancer*
Whole-grain muffin with fruit jam (optional)

LUNCH
Vegetable stir-fry on rice
Beverage
Dessert (optional)

DINNER
Grilled tuna steak with leeks
Sautéed Greens with Sesame Seeds*
Warm beverage

Recommended Beverages

Green tea
Herb teas
Fresh fruit and vegetable juices
Water
Soy milk
Rice milk
Coffee substitutes
Organic coffee
Hormone-free milk

BREATHING AND EXERCISE PLAN

Note: It takes time to combine diaphragmatic breathing and exercise. When learning, stay with the exercises at Level 1. When you move to Level 2, start with metabolic breathing. Only when you have mastered metabolic breathing should you go on to Level 3.

Start-up

Practice ten minutes of diaphragmatic breathing daily. Then begin to incorporate it into your day by setting a timer or beeper to go off so that you can breathe diaphragmatically *every* hour. In three weeks you'll forget how you used to breathe.

When comfortable with diaphragmatic breathing, combine it with exercises. Then move on to the metabolic breathing method.

Optional Exercises

1. Practice alternate-nostril breathing for five minutes in the morning and five minutes in the evening.

2. After you've mastered metabolic breathing, try doing bellows for fifteen to thirty seconds before exercising. (Make sure you have an empty stomach.)

Exercise Sequences
(Fifteen to Twenty-five Minutes)

LEVEL 1	LEVEL 2	LEVEL 3
1. Body-Scanning Technique	Body-Scanning Technique	Body-Scanning Technique
2. Celestial Breath	Hip Circles	Hip Circles
3. Windmills	Standing Cat with a Turn	Standing Cat with a Turn
4. Standing Cat with a Turn	Woodchopper	Woodchopper
5. The Turtle	The Lunge	The Lunge
6. Wood Chopper	The Squat	The Squat
7. Hip Circles	Pike Position	Pike Position
8. Single Straight Lifts	Double Lifts	Double Lifts
9. Hip Releaser	Energy Pump	Around the World
10. The Twist	Hip Releaser	Metabolic Master
11. Rocking	Pretzel Twist	Metabolic Master II
12. Pelvic Lift I	Pelvic Lift II	Pelvic Lift II
13. Body Scanning	Body Scanning	Body Scanning

Note: These are basic sequences to start. You may like one exercise more than others. The sequence is designed to work all the body parts. First become familiar with them, then you can tailor your own workout.

RECIPES FOR THE VITALITY DIET

Note: You may make substitutions in all recipes—for example, use grapefruit juice instead of lemon juice. For ease, you can use precooked beans and frozen fruits and vegetables as substitutes for fresh foods, but avoid canned foods entirely. Many of the dishes are available at salad bars and restaurants. The emphasis is to follow the basic format and eat as many healthy foods as possible.

Day 1

SEXUAL REJUVENATOR

Juice of 1 large lemon (or 2 small)
4–6 oz. spring water (room temperature)
1–2 tsp. honey or unsulfered molasses

Combine ingredients and drink.

Alternative: Use half the amount of lemon juice and add a pinch of cayenne pepper.

METABOLIC CLEANSER

Juice of $^1/_2$ medium grapefruit
Juice of 1 medium orange
1 tsp. lemon juice
$^1/_4$ cup frozen blueberries or 1 banana

Combine ingredients in a blender for 15 seconds and serve.

FLAXSEED CEREAL WITH SOY MILK

$^1/_3$ cup dried oats
1 cup soy milk
1 tsp. ground flaxseed
$^1/_3$ cup berries or cut fruit

1. Place oats in warm iron skillet and keep turning over medium heat until golden brown.
2. Remove oats from skillet and place in medium saucepan with soy milk. Bring to a boil over high heat.
3. Reduce heat to low. Cover and cook until desired consistency, 2–5 minutes.

4. Add flaxseed and let stand for 3 minutes.
5. Add fruit and serve.

BAKED FALAFEL

4 cups dried chickpeas that have been soaked overnight in 3 cups water and drained
2 tsp. cumin
1 tsp. turmeric
1 tsp. sea salt
6 scallions, minced
$1/4$ cup parsley, chopped
$1/4$ cup water
1 tbsp. lemon juice
1 tbsp. olive oil
$1/2$ cup flour

1. Preheat oven to 350 degrees.
2. Coat a baking sheet with olive oil and heat in oven for 10 minutes.
3. Place all ingredients except flour in a food processor and combine at medium speed for 10 seconds.
4. Form mixture in patties about $3 1/2$ inches in diameter and $2/3$ inch thick.
5. Coat patties lightly with flour and place on hot baking sheet. Bake 10 minutes on each side.

MIXED STEAMED GREENS

2 lbs. Russian kale
2 lbs. collards
2 lbs. Swiss chard
1 tbsp. olive oil
3–4 cloves garlic, chopped
1 leek, chopped
$1/2$ cup water

1. Wash all greens. Do not dry. Chop fine.
2. Heat large skillet or wok over medium heat.
3. Add oil and sauté garlic and leek.
4. Add greens and toss. Sprinkle greens with just enough water to keep from sticking to the pot. Cover and cook on low heat until greens are tender, 3–5 minutes.
5. Turn off the heat and let sit for 5 minutes in the covered pot. Serve.

Day 2

HORMONE BALANCER

1 cup vanilla soy milk
1–2 tbsp. soy powder
¹/₂ frozen banana
Juice of 2 oranges

Combine ingredients in a blender for 15 seconds. Serve cold.

RICE CEREAL WITH SOY MILK
(AN ALTERNATIVE TO OATMEAL)

1 cup cooked basmati rice
¹/₄–¹/₃ tsp. cinnamon
¹/₄ cup ginger (optional)
1 cup soy milk
2 tbsp. honey or maple syrup

1. Put rice, cinnamon, ginger (if desired), and soy milk in small saucepan and mix well.
2. Cook over medium heat, about 5 minutes.
3. Add honey (or maple syrup) and serve.

WILD-RICE SALAD

¹/₂ cup wild rice with ¹/₄ cup rice blend
2 cups prepackaged vegetable stock

1–2 cups chopped kale and/or spinach
2 scallions, chopped

1. Cook rice as indicated using vegetable stock as liquid.
2. Add greens and scallions for the last 15 minutes of cooking time. Serve immediately.

ROASTED RICE

1 cup long-grain brown rice
2 cups water or vegetarian vegetable stock
Pinch of sea salt (optional)

1. Put rice in an iron skillet over high heat. Stir until kernels are lightly browned.
2. Add water or stock and salt. Bring to a boil and cover.
3. Reduce heat to medium low and simmer until water is absorbed.
4. Remove from heat and let stand for 5–10 minutes, covered.
5. Remove lid and serve.

Day 3

FRESH FRUIT PLATE WITH GRANOLA TOPPING

1/2 pineapple, cubed
1–2 kiwis
1 banana
1/4 cup granola (see below)

Cut fruits into bite-sized pieces. Add topping and serve.

GRANOLA

4–5 cups oats (avoid quick oats)
1 cup sweetener (honey, maple syrup, molasses)
1/4 cup chopped pecans
1/4 cup sunflower seeds

$^1/_2$ *cup chopped dates (optional)*
2 *tbsp. flaxseeds (optional)*

1. Preheat oven to 300 degrees.
2. Mix all ingredients and put on a baking sheet.
3. Cook until golden brown or to the dryness you like, stirring every 5 minutes. Let cool.
4. Store in a tight jar and refrigerate.

TOASTED OATS

$^1/_3$ *cup dried oats*
1 *cup water or milk*
$^1/_8$ *tsp. cinnamon*
Pinch of ginger (optional)
Ghee, honey, or maple sugar (optional)

1. Place the oats in a warm iron skillet and toast over medium heat until golden brown.
2. Remove oats from skillet and place in a medium saucepan with milk or water. Bring to a boil.
3. Reduce heat to low. Add cinnamon and ginger. Cook until desired consistency, 5–10 minutes. Add ghee, honey, or maple sugar to taste.

PIZZA LINGUINE STYLE

$^1/_2$ *chopped onion*
2–3 *cloves garlic*
1 *tbsp. fennel seeds*
1 *tbsp. olive oil*
1 *cup chopped mushrooms*
$^1/_2$ *cup chopped eggplant*
$^1/_2$ *cup chopped zucchini*
$1^1/_2$ *cups tomato sauce (use your favorite fat-free, sugar-free variety)*
$^1/_2$–1 *cup cubed tofu*

1 tbsp. oregano
8–10 oz. pasta

1. Preheat oven to 375 degrees.
2. Sauté onions, garlic, and fennel seeds in olive oil. Set aside.
3. Combine the rest of the ingredients (except pasta) in a medium saucepan and simmer for 15–20 minutes over low heat.
4. Cook pasta in separate pot. Drain and put in casserole dish.
5. Add vegetable mixture on top of pasta. Bake for 25 minutes.

ENERGY SALAD

3 cups romaine lettuce or other leaf lettuce, such as radicchio, water-cress, or Boston
1–2 organic tomatoes, sliced
1 carrot, sliced
1 cucumber, sliced

Combine ingredients and serve with one of the dressings below.

OLIVE OIL/GARLIC DRESSING

1 tbsp. olive oil
2 cloves garlic, minced
Juice of $1/_2$ lemon
Pinch of cayenne pepper (optional)

Combine ingredients in a jar and shake vigorously.

CLASSIC VINAIGRETTE DRESSING

1 tbsp. olive oil or other oil, such as canola, sesame, or walnut
2 tbsps. vinegar

Note: For variety, add minced garlic, mustard, fresh herbs such as basil, honey, or brown-rice syrup. Experiment for yourself.

Combine in a jar and shake vigorously.

Day 4

VITALITY PROMOTER

4 large carrots
1 large red beet (or 2 medium)
2 stalks celery
10 parsley sprigs
2 collard or kale leaves
Juice of 1 lemon

1. Place carrots, beets, celery, parsley, and greens in a juicer.
2. Add the lemon juice.
3. Mix and serve.

PHYTOESTROGEN DELIGHT

1 lb. tofu, cubed
1–2 tsp. turmeric
1–2 tbsp. mustard
Protein powder (optional)
1 green pepper, chopped
1 scallion, chopped

1. In food processor or bowl, add tofu, turmeric, mustard, and protein powder. Blend well for 10 seconds.
2. Hand-mix in green pepper and scallion. Serve.

Day 5

PASTA PESTO

2–3 cups basil leaves, washed and dried
³/₄ cup olive oil
1 tsp. fine sea salt
1 tbsp. lemon juice (optional)
¹/₂ cup grated Parmesan cheese (optional)
Freshly ground black pepper

$^1/_4$ *cup toasted whole pine nuts (use unsalted pistachio nuts for a*
  lower-fat substitute)

1. Combine all ingredients except pine nuts in a food processor. Blend for 15 seconds.
2. Add pine nuts by folding them in.
3. Refrigerate before serving. For later use, store in freezer.

MINERAL MOUNTAIN

1 qt. water
1 cup wakama
1 cup cubed tofu
1 tbsp. shredded kornbu
1 scallion, chopped
1 carrot, chopped
1–2 tbsp. miso paste
Tamari to taste (optional)

1. In saucepan, combine all ingredients except miso paste and tamari.
2. Bring to a boil and let simmer for 10 minutes.
3. In separate cup put miso and add $^1/_4$–$^1/_2$ cup of soup mixture to dissolve. Let stand for 5 minutes.
4. Add miso mixture to saucepan.
5. Add tamari to taste and serve.

STUFFED ZUCCHINI

4 medium zucchini
1 tbsp. olive oil
1 small onion, chopped
1 beaten egg or 2 beaten egg whites
1 cup chopped tofu
1 tsp. cayenne pepper
1 dash nutmeg
1 tsp. unrefined sea salt

$^1/_2$ *cup whole-grain bread crumbs*
$^1/_4$ *tsp. sweet paprika*

1. Preheat oven to 350 degrees.
2. Cut zucchini lengthwise. Scoop out inside and chop. Place in medium-sized bowl.
3. In skillet, heat olive oil and sauté onion until soft. Add to bowl with zucchini seeds.
4. In same skillet, sauté zucchini on both sides over medium heat until lightly brown.
5. Add beaten egg, tofu, cayenne, nutmeg, salt, and bread crumbs to onion mixture. Mix thoroughly.
6. Divide stuffing among eight halves.
7. Sprinkle paprika on top.
8. Bake for 20–25 minutes.

Day 6

BANANA SOY SHAKE

1–2 frozen bananas
$^1/_2$ *cup organic strawberries or other berries in season*
2 cups vanilla soy milk

Combine the ingredients in a blender. Mix until desired consistency.

SWEET FRUIT SALAD

$^1/_2$ *cup pineapple cubes*
$^1/_2$ *cup blueberries*
1 sliced banana
1 tbsp. honey
3 tbsp. chopped blanched almonds

Combine fruit in a bowl. Mix honey and almonds and dribble on top.

VEGETABLE BEAN PIE

2–3 tbsp. water
2 large tomatoes, sliced
2 zucchini, cubed
1 cup sliced mushrooms
½–1 cup cubed tofu
1 onion, finely chopped
2–3 cloves garlic, finely chopped
1 cup vegetable broth (reconstituted from a powder)
½ cup uncooked brown rice
3 egg whites, well blended
1–2 cups cooked garbanzo beans (chickpeas), rinsed and drained
1 tsp. fresh basil
1 tsp. olive oil

1. Preheat oven to 350 degrees.
2. Place water in a saucepan and bring to boil. Add tomatoes, zucchini, mushrooms, tofu, onion, and garlic. Steam approximately 5 minutes. Uncover and let stand.
3. In another saucepan, bring vegetable broth to a boil. Add rice and return to boil. Then lower heat and cook until water is absorbed.
4. Add egg whites, beans, and basil to the rice.
5. Cover the bottom of a baking dish with olive oil to prevent sticking and then spread the rice mixture.
6. Add the vegetable and tofu mixture on top of the rice. Bake 20–25 minutes.

HUMMUS SPREAD

2 cups cooked chickpeas
⅔ (approximately) cup bean liquid
2 tbsp. lemon juice
2 scallions, chopped (optional)
2–3 cloves garlic

3 tbsp. tahini (sesame butter)
$\frac{1}{2}$ tsp. sea salt

1. Soak one cup of dry chickpeas overnight.
2. Boil the chickpeas in a covered pot for 3–4 hours or until they mash easily between your fingers. Drain well and save the liquid.
3. Put the beans, lemon juice, scallions, and garlic in a blender or food processor with just enough liquid from the beans to blend.
4. Add the tahini and salt, and mix well. Note: Tahini will thicken the mixture, so adjust the consistency with additional liquid from the beans.

THYROID BALANCER (KELP SOUP)

4 cups water
6-inch piece of kelp
2 carrots, finely chopped
1 cup collard greens, finely chopped
Miso
Tamari (optional)

1. In a saucepan, combine all ingredients except miso and tamari.
2. Bring to a boil and let simmer for 10 minutes.
3. In a separate cup put miso and dissolve with $\frac{1}{4}$–$\frac{1}{2}$ cup of soup mixture. Let stand for 5 minutes.
4. Turn off heat under saucepan.
5. Add miso mixture to saucepan. Let stand for 5 minutes.
6. Add tamari to taste and serve.

Day 7

FATIGUE ELIMINATOR

7 sprigs of parsley
1 cucumber

1 large red beet or two medium beets
4 large carrots
Juice of $1/2$–1 lemon
Cayenne pepper (optional)

In a juicer, add parsley and cucumber, followed by beets and carrots. Add the lemon juice and a pinch of cayenne if desired. Drink immediately.

LENTIL SOUP

1 lb. dry lentils
7–8 cups water
6–8 cloves garlic, minced
1 medium onion, chopped
2 stalks celery, chopped
2 carrots, chopped
1 tbsp. pesto (optional; see recipe, Day 5)
8 oz. tomato sauce or 2 large tomatoes pureed in food processor
   (optional)
Sea salt to taste
Freshly ground black pepper
Brown-rice vinegar

1. Wash and drain lentils.
2. Place in pot with water. Bring to a boil.
3. Add garlic, onion, celery, and carrots.
4. Add pesto and tomatoes if desired.
5. Reduce heat to simmer and cook until lentils are soft, approximately 1 hour.
6. Drizzle brown-rice vinegar on top. Sprinkle with black pepper.
7. Serve with crisp bread.

ASPARAGUS WITH HONEY-LEMON DRESSING

$3/4$ cup tahini or peanut butter
6 tbsp. lemon juice
1 tbsp. honey

2 tbsp. minced garlic
3/4 cup or more water
1/2 tsp. fine sea salt
Pinch of cayenne pepper to taste
Fresh parsley (optional)
1 1/4 lbs. fresh asparagus
1 tsp. olive oil

1. Preheat oven to 350 degrees.
2. Place tahini or peanut butter, lemon juice, honey, and minced garlic in food processor. Add water and blend until desired consistency. Add salt, cayenne, and parsley.
3. Chop off tough ends of asparagus. Put in baking dish. Drizzle with olive oil. Spoon dressing over asparagus. Cover and bake for 15 minutes or until asparagus is tender.

Day 8

STUFFED EGGPLANT

3 medium eggplant
1 tbsp. extra-virgin olive oil
1 small onion, chopped
8 oz. chopped mushrooms
2 cups cooked brown rice
1 tbsp. pesto (see recipe, Day 5)
1/2 cup grated Parmesan cheese or cubed tofu
1 cup tomato sauce (use your favorite organic variety)
1 tsp. refined sea salt (optional)
Dash of thyme
Dash of oregano
Freshly ground black pepper
4 large cloves garlic, minced
1 handful fresh parsley

1. Preheat oven to 350 degrees.
2. Cut eggplant in half lengthwise and scoop out the insides, leaving a 1/8-inch shell. Cut the flesh into 1/2-inch cubes.

3. Heat olive oil in skillet. Sauté onion and mushrooms until soft. Add rice, pesto, cheese or tofu, tomato sauce, sea salt, thyme, oregano, and pepper. Cook 3 minutes.
4. Add chopped garlic and parsley.
5. Divide the ingredients into 6 parts and stuff shells.
6. Bake for 30 minutes.

GRILLED SHRIMP, MUSHROOMS, AND SNOW PEAS ON A BED OF RICE

2 tbsp. olive or sesame oil
2 lbs. cleaned shrimp
3 cloves garlic, minced
1 lb. mushrooms
$^1/_2$ lb. snow peas
1 tsp. low-sodium tamari (optional)
2 cups cooked basmati rice

1. In a large skillet or wok, heat oil and sauté shrimp 3–5 minutes. Remove to a side plate.
2. Add garlic to skillet and sauté until light brown.
3. Add mushrooms and snow peas and toss for approximately 3 minutes.
4. Add shrimp and lightly toss.
5. Add tamari. Serve on bed of basmati rice.

Day 9

PASTA WITH TOFU AND TOMATO PESTO SAUCE

3 lbs. plum tomatoes
1 tbsp. olive oil
2 large cloves garlic
$^1/_2$ tsp. fennel seeds
1 tbsp. pesto (see recipe, Day 5)
2 cups cubed tofu
1 lb. fusilli, penne, shells, or other pasta

1. Puree tomatoes in a food processor. Empty into 4-qt. pot.
2. Heat oil in a skillet. Add garlic and fennel seeds and sauté until garlic is soft.
3. Add garlic and fennel mixture to tomatoes. Add pesto and cook $1/2$ hour or until thickened.
4. Ten minutes before done, add the cubed tofu.
5. Pour over cooked pasta and serve.

GARLICKY GREENS

2 lbs. leafy greens, such as spinach, Swiss chard, dandelion, kale, collards, bok choy
2 tbsp. extra-virgin olive oil or toasted sesame oil
5 large cloves garlic, chopped
1 leek, chopped
1 tbsp. sesame seeds
$1/2$ tsp. tamari

1. Clean all greens. If using kale, collards, or spinach, remove the stems.
2. In a large wok or heavy skillet, heat oil over low heat. Do not let oil smoke. Add garlic and leek and sauté until garlic is light brown.
3. Add greens and stir-fry for about 3 minutes. Add sesame seeds and stir-fry until leaves are tender.
4. Remove from heat. Add tamari and cover for about 2 minutes. Serve.

Day 10

TABOULEH

1 cup bulgur wheat, rinsed
$1^3/4$ cups boiling water
$1/4$ cup lemon juice
$1/4$ cup extra-virgin olive oil

2 cloves garlic, minced

1/4 tsp. cayenne pepper (optional)

Sea salt to taste

2 large ripe tomatoes

1 large cucumber, chopped

4 scallions, chopped

1/3 cup chopped cilentro or Italian parsley

10 chopped mint leaves (optional)

1. Combine bulgur and water in large mixing bowl. Let stand until bulgur is tender, for about 10 minutes.
2. Drain.
3. Add lemon juice, olive oil, garlic, cayenne, and sea salt.
4. Refrigerate for at least 1 hour, then add remaining ingredients and mix well. Serve.

MARINATED TOFU

1 lb. tofu

1 tbsp. tamari or soy sauce

1 tsp. mirin

3 scallions, chopped

1 large clove garlic, minced

1 tbsp. toasted sesame oil

1 tbsp. kuzu (thickener)

1 tbsp. toasted sesame seeds

1. Cut tofu into 1/2-inch slices and place in a saucepan.
2. Add tamari, mirin, scallions, and garlic and marinate for 1/2 hour.
3. Remove tofu from marinade and drain.
4. In a skillet, heat oil. Add tofu and grill for about 5 minutes on each side.
5. Bring the marinade to a boil and add kuzu to dissolve. Simmer for 1–3 minutes or until thickened.
6. Pour over tofu. Sprinkle with sesame seeds and serve.

Day 11

SEA VEGETABLE SALAD

1 cup dried hijiki
1½ cup dried arama
½ cup chopped carrots
3 scallions, chopped
½ lb. tofu, cubed
1 tbsp. toasted sesame seeds

DRESSING

½ cup wheat-free tamari
½ cup hot pepper sesame oil
½ cup brown-rice vinegar
½ cup marin

1. Wash hijiki and arama in a collander for about 5 minutes. Then let soak in fresh water for ½ hour. Drain.
2. Bring 4 qts. of water to boil and add sea vegetables.
3. Simmer on low heat for approximately 30 minutes or until tender.
4. Drain and let cool.
5. Meanwhile make dressing.
6. Add carrots, scallions, tofu, sesame seeds, and dressing to sea vegetables.
7. Toss and let stand for 30 minutes before serving.

Day 12

SWISS CHARD PIZZA

Rolled pizza dough
Dash of cornmeal
2 lbs. Swiss chard
1 tbsp. olive oil

2 cloves garlic, minced
$^1/_4$ cup grated Parmesan cheese (optional)
20 pitted Kalamata olives
$^1/_4$ cup shredded mozzarella

1. Preheat oven to 375 degrees.
2. Place rolled dough in oiled baking pan and sprinkle with cornmeal.
3. Wash chard and leave damp.
4. Heat oil in skillet and sauté garlic until light brown.
5. Add chard and sauté until tender. Spread on dough.
6. Sprinkle with Parmesan and arrange pitted olives. Add mozzarella.
7. Bake for 40 minutes and serve.

CHICKPEAS IN HOT TOMATO SAUCE

2 cups dried chickpeas
6 cups water for cooking
1 qt. tomato sauce (use your favorite organic variety)

1. Soak chickpeas overnight in 3 cups of water.
2. Drain and add 6 cups of fresh water. Bring to a boil, then simmer for about 3 hours or until tender (you may have to add more water). Drain.
3. Add tomato sauce and simmer for 20 minutes. Cover and let stand for 15 minutes before serving.

TOMATO/BASIL/FENNEL SAUCE

3 lbs. ripe plum tomatoes
1 tsp. olive oil
1 tsp. minced garlic
1 tsp. fennel seeds
1 tbsp. pesto (see recipe, Day 5) or handful of basil leaves
2 cayenne peppers (optional)

1. In food processor, chop tomatoes.
2. Heat oil in skillet and sauté garlic and fennel until garlic is light brown. Add to chopped tomatoes.
4. Add pesto or basil and cayenne.
5. Simmer until thick, 30–40 minutes.

Day 13

FRUIT SMOOTHIE

1 frozen banana
2 oranges
1 cup organic frozen strawberries or other berries
1 cup vanilla soy milk
1 tbsp. protein powder (optional)

1. Place all ingredients in a blender.
2. Mix at high speed for 20 seconds and serve.

LENTIL SALAD IN PITA BREAD

4 cups water
2 cups dried rinsed lentils
1 bay leaf
³/₄ cup diced red onion
1 clove garlic, minced
¹/₂ cup diced carrots
¹/₂ cup any vegetable of your choice (optional)
6-inch strip kombu (sea vegetable)

1. In 4-qt. pot, add water, lentils, and bay leaf. Cover and heat to boil.
2. After 10 minutes, add onion, garlic, carrots, chopped vegetables, and kombu.
3. Uncover and continue to boil until lentils are tender, 20–45 minutes.

DRESSING

$^1/_2$ *cup extra-virgin olive oil*
2 tbsp. lemon juice or vinegar
1$^1/_2$ tsp. Dijon mustard
2 cloves garlic, minced

1. Place all ingredients in small jar and shake vigorously to blend.
2. Let stand for at least 1 hour before using.
3. Refrigerate unused portion.
4. Pour dressing over salad and serve on pita bread.

Day 14

EGGLESS TOFU

1 lb. fat-reduced tofu
2 tbsp. tahini
4 tbsp. protein powder (optional)
2 tbsp. onions, chopped
$^1/_2$ *green pepper, chopped (optional)*
$^1/_2$ *tsp. cayenne pepper*
$^1/_2$ *tsp. garlic powder or 2 cloves fresh garlic, chopped*
$^1/_4$ *tsp. turmeric*
1 tbsp. Dijon mustard
1 stalk celery, chopped

Mash the tofu with a fork. Add the remaining ingredients and mix by hand. If you prefer smoother consistency, use a blender.

RATATOUILLE OVER RICE

1 tsp. olive oil
5 cloves garlic
1 tbsp. fennel seeds
1 large onion

2 cups mushrooms (optional)
3 medium zucchini, cubed
2 bell peppers, chopped
1 eggplant, cubed
6–8 okra, chopped
2 cups fresh tomato sauce (see recipe, Day 9)

1. Heat oil in large skillet and sauté garlic, fennel, onion, and mushrooms.
2. In a large pot, add zucchini, peppers, eggplant, and okra. Cook over medium heat to get some of the water out of the vegetables, stirring constantly, approximately 15 minutes.
3. Add tomato sauce and sautéed vegetables. Simmer and cook for 25 minutes.
4. Turn off heat and let stand for 15 minutes before serving.

CUCUMBER SALAD WITH VINAIGRETTE

3 cucumbers, peeled and cubed
3 tbsp. oil
1 tbsp. vinegar
1 clove garlic
Dash oregano or thyme

1. Put cucumber in a mixing bowl.
2. Mix remaining ingredients. Pour over cucumbers and toss.
3. Let stand 30 minutes before serving.

Day 15

EGG-WHITE OMELET WITH MUSHROOMS AND TOFU

1 egg
5 egg whites
1 tbsp. olive oil
1 green pepper, diced (optional)
1 small zucchini

$^1/_2$ cup chopped mushrooms
$^1/_4$ cup tofu, cubed
3 scallions (optional)
1 tsp. hing (aids digestion)

1. Combine egg and egg whites in a bowl and stir with a fork until well blended.
2. Heat oil in saucepan and sauté remaining ingredients.
3. Add egg mixture. Cover and cook over low flame for approximately 10 minutes or until eggs are cooked thoroughly.
4. Remove from heat and serve.

SAUTÉED BRUSSELS SPROUTS

2 cups brussels sprouts, washed and cleaned
1 tsp. olive oil
2 cloves garlic, minced
1 tsp. fennel seeds
Dash of tamari

1. Steam brussels sprouts until cooked but not soft.
2. Heat oil in a skillet and sauté garlic with fennel seeds until garlic is light brown.
3. Add brussels sprouts and tamari. Cover and cook over medium heat for 5 minutes.

Day 16

VEGETABLE–APPLE JUICE COCKTAIL

4–5 carrots
1 apple
1 stalk celery

Place ingredients in juicer and mix.

ZUCCHINI BREAD

3 cups flour
2 tsp. cinnamon
2 tsp. baking powder
1 tsp. baking soda
3 cups grated zucchini
3 beaten eggs (or 5 egg whites)
1/2 cup raw sugar
1/4 cup vegetable oil
1 cup walnuts

1. Preheat oven to 325 degrees.
2. Mix flour, cinnamon, baking powder, and baking soda in a small mixing bowl.
3. Combine zucchini, eggs, sugar, and oil in a large mixing bowl and beat with fork or whisk until well blended.
4. Add the flour mixture to the zucchini-egg mixture. Add the walnuts and mix well.
5. Empty into loaf pan and bake 1 hour.

COLD PASTA SALAD WITH TOMATO, BASIL, AND TOFU

1/2 lb. pasta of choice (e.g., fusilli, penne, shells)
2 cloves garlic, minced
1/2 lb. firm tofu, cubed
15 fresh basil leaves
3–4 large beefsteak tomatoes, cubed
2 tbsp. olive oil
Black pepper to taste

1. Prepare pasta.
2. While pasta is cooking, in large bowl mix garlic, tofu, basil, tomatoes, and olive oil. Add pepper.
3. Mix pasta with tomato-basil mixture and refrigerate.

Day 17

TOFU CHICKEN SALAD

1 lb. fat-reduced tofu
2 tbsp. tahini
4 tbsp. nutritional yeast
2 tbsp. shallots or onions, chopped
1/2 tsp. cayenne pepper
1/4 tsp. garlic powder or 2 cloves fresh garlic, chopped
1/4 tsp. celery seeds
1 tsp. barbecue seasoning or tamari (optional)
1 stalk celery, chopped
1–3 tbsp. spring water (optional)

1. Put tofu in a bowl and break apart with fork.
2. Add remaining ingredients and mix. Depending on desired consistency, use a blender. If too dry, add 1–3 tablespoons of spring water.

STIR-FRIED GREENS WITH GINGER

1 lb. greens, such as spinach, Swiss chard, dandelion, kale, collards, bok choy
1 tbsp. hot sesame oil
5 slices fresh ginger
1 leek

1. Wash all greens. Do not dry.
2. Heat oil in a large skillet or wok. Add ginger and leek and sauté until light brown.
3. Add greens and toss. Cover and cook over medium heat for 5–10 minutes or until greens are tender.

Day 18

GARDEN BURGER

1 lb. tofu
1 tbsp. olive oil

1 large onion
1 large clove garlic
1 tsp. cumin
1 cup tomato sauce (use your favorite organic variety)
1 tsp. unrefined sea salt (optional)
$\frac{1}{2}$ cup toasted almonds, ground
Black pepper to taste
1 cup whole-wheat bread crumbs

1. Preheat oven to 350 degrees.
2. In a large mixing bowl, mash tofu with fork. Set aside.
3. Heat oil in skillet. Add onion, garlic, and cumin and sauté until light brown.
4. Add tomato sauce and salt and simmer for 5–10 minutes.
5. Pour this mixture into bowl with tofu. Mix.
6. Add nuts and mix. Add pepper if desired.
7. Cool mixture. Add bread crumbs and form into patties, about $3\frac{1}{2}$ inches in diameter and $\frac{2}{3}$ inch thick. Use extra bread crumbs if needed.
8. Bake on a lightly oiled baking sheet approximately 10 minutes on each side or until crispy.

MARINATED SHRIMP AND CHICKEN KEBOBS
WITH GRILLED VEGETABLES

1 lb. raw shrimp
1 lb. boneless and skinless chicken
1 zucchini, cut into $\frac{1}{2}$-inch slices
1 yellow squash, cut into $\frac{1}{2}$-inch slices
1 mushroom
1 green pepper, cut into 1-inch pieces
1 red pepper, cut into 1-inch pieces

Prepare marinade:

$\frac{1}{4}$ cup olive oil
$\frac{1}{8}$ cup vinegar

1 clove garlic, minced
dash oregano

1. Combine the marinade ingredients and pour into two separate bowls.
2. Clean and devein shrimp. Cut up chicken into ¾-inch pieces.
3. Marinate chicken in one bowl and shrimp in the other for 1 hour.
4. Put on skewers with vegetables.
5. Barbecue or cook under broiler until golden.

Day 19

LIGHT VEGETABLE BROTH

2 large potatoes, diced
4 carrots, chopped
4 stalks celery, chopped
5 cloves garlic, minced
2 leeks
3 large bay leaves
2 cups chopped mixed vegetables (peas, broccoli stalks, green beans)
Dash of parsley (optional)
2 cups tomato sauce (optional; see recipe, Day 9)
5 cups water

1. Combine all ingredients in a large pot and bring to a boil.
2. Reduce heat and simmer for 1 hour.
3. Let stand for 30 minutes.
4. Press vegetables through strainer.
5. Let cool and refrigerate. Good for a maximum of 2 days in refrigerator, or up to 6 weeks in freezer.

TEMPEH VEGETABLE STIR-FRY

1 tbsp. toasted sesame oil
1 tbsp. grated fresh ginger

1 leek, chopped
1 package tempeh, cubed
1 cayenne pepper (optional)
2 large carrots, chopped
4 cups chopped washed greens, such as spinach, Swiss chard, dandelion, kale, collards, bok choy
Tamari to taste

1. Heat oil in large skillet or wok and lightly sauté ginger and leek.
2. Turn down flame and add tempeh and cayenne. Sauté until tempeh is golden.
3. Add carrots and greens and toss.
4. Cover and cook over medium heat until carrots and greens are tender. Sprinkle with water if pan is too dry.
5. Serve with tamari.

Day 20

COUSCOUS SALAD

1 cup couscous
2 cups boiling water or seasoned vegetable broth (prepackaged)
1 tbsp. olive oil
1 clove garlic, minced
3 scallions, minced
2 carrots, chopped
$1/2$ cup thawed frozen peas
2 cups asparagus spears, chopped

1. Place couscous in a large serving bowl. Add boiling water or vegetable broth and stir. Cover and let sit for 10 minutes or until water is absorbed.
2. Meanwhile heat oil in a large wok or skillet. Add garlic and scallions and sauté. Add vegetables. Stir-fry until vegetables are tender.
3. Spread vegetables on top of couscous and serve.

Day 21

SAUTÉED GREENS WITH SESAME SEEDS

1 lb. greens, such as spinach, Swiss chard, dandelion, kale, collards, bok choy
1 tbsp. hot sesame oil
5 slices fresh ginger
2 cloves garlic, minced
3 scallions, chopped
1 tbsp. dry roasted sesame seeds
Tamari to taste

1. Wash all greens. Do not dry.
2. Heat oil in a large skillet or wok. Add ginger, garlic, and scallions and sauté lightly.
3. Add greens and toss. Cover and let steam for 5–10 minutes or until greens are tender.
4. Add sesame seeds and tamari. Toss and let stand for 3 minutes before serving.

APPENDICES

$\mathcal{V}$ITALITY DIET FOOD GUIDE

BEANS
Black
Chickpeas
Great Northern
Kidney
Lentil
Lima
Mung
Pinto
Soy
Split peas

SOY PRODUCTS
Miso
Tempeh
Tofu

WHOLE GRAINS
Barley
Basmati rice
Brown rice
Couscous, whole wheat
Millet
Oatmeal, pretoasted
Quinoa
Rice cakes
Whole-grain crackers
Wild rice

FRUIT
Apricots
Avocados
Bananas
Berries
Dates
Figs
Grapefruit
Lemons
Melons
Oranges
Peaches

VEGETABLES
Artichokes
Asparagus
Beets
Broccoli
Brussels sprouts
Cabbage, red and green
Carrots
Celery
Collards
Cucumbers
Dandelion greens
Endive
Escarole
Green beans
Kale
Leeks
Lettuce, all leafy varieties
Mushrooms
Mustard greens
Onions
Shallots

NUTS AND SEEDS
Almonds
Cashews
Flaxseeds
Pecans
Pumpkin seeds
Sesame seeds
Sunflower seeds
Walnuts

CONDIMENTS AND OILS
All fruit jams
Apple cider vinegar
Barley malt
Brown-rice syrup

Brown-rice vinegar
Peanut butter
Tahini
Canola oil
Cold-pressed sesame oil
Extra-virgin olive oil
Peanut oil

SPICES AND HERBS
Basil
Cinnamon
Cloves
Coriander
Cumin
Fennel
Garlic
Ginger
Hing
Nutmeg
Rosemary
Turmeric

SEA VEGETABLES
Agar-agar
Arame
Dulse
Hijiki
Kelp
Komby
Nori
Shiitake
Wakame

BEVERAGES
Green tea
Herbal teas
Kukicha tea

$\mathscr{C}$OMMON ESSENTIAL OILS (NOT TO BE INGESTED)

Basil: One of the best aromatic nerve tonics. Use to relieve mental fatigue due to stress.

Chamomile: Relieves stress by relaxing the body and calming the nerves.

Clary Sage: Use as a tonic for nervous system.

Cypress: Astringent. Use in combination with juniper to tone muscles.

Jasmine: Traditionally used as an aphrodisiac. Elevates mood, relaxes, and induces euphoria.

Juniper: One of the most versatile of oils. Has many properties, one being a diuretic. Use in combination with cypress to help decrease cellulite.

Lavender: Relieves stress and helps relieve headaches.

Neroli: Among the finest in flower essences. Acts to renew cells. Makes a luxurious and relaxing bath or massage oil.

Rose: The quintessential scent of romance. Stimulates sexual responsiveness and feelings of sensuality.

Rosemary: Nervous-system stimulant. Produces clarity of mind.

Sandlewood: Use to relax and calm the mind and body. Excellent when combined with other oils.

Ylang-Ylang: Aphrodisiac. Called the flower of flowers. One of the most emotionally evocative essential oils.

ESSENTIAL OIL RECIPES

THIGH ENHANCER
Juniper (1–2 drops in bath), cypress (1–2 drops in bath), and lavender (2 drops in bath). Those troubled with cellulite due to fluid retention will find this useful and relaxing.

TENSION RELIEVER
Lavender. One drop on temples will relieve headache due to stress. A few drops on pillow aids sleep.

STRESS BUSTER
Neroli (3 drops in bath). Eases tension and stress. Aids in sleep. Mixes well with lavender.

MENTAL REJUVENATOR
Juniper, rosemary, and basil. Mix 5 drops of each in 30 ml. of oil. Massage on temples to promote alertness.

SENSUALITY STIMULANT
Ylang-Ylang. As a massage oil, must be diluted, so add 5 drops to 10 ml. oil. As a bath oil, add 4 drops to 2 drops of sandlewood.

MENSTRUAL PAIN RELIEVER
Lavender (4 drops), chamomile (3 drops), and clary sage (3 drops). Mix in 10 ml. almond oil. Rub over abdomen and lower back.

*F*LOWER ESSENCES FOR SEXUAL VITALITY

Aloe Vera: Use to rejuvenate the body and redirect creative forces.

Alpine Lily: Enhances vital female energy.

Arnica: Repairs life energy after shock or trauma.

California Wild Rose: Overcomes apathy.

Crab Apple: Eases feelings of shame.

Easter Lily: Relieves menopause toxicity.

Evening Primrose: Helps reconnect with intimacy.

Hibiscus: Helps connect with one's female sexuality.

Lady's Slipper: Helps with sexual depletion. Balances lower chakras.

Maripose Lily: Helps relieve trauma of childhood sexual abuse.

Morning Glory: Revitalizes energy.

Mountain Pride: Stimulates assertiveness.

Olive: Reinvigorates energy after physical exertion.

Pink Monkey Flower: Eases feelings of unworthiness and shame.

Pretty Face: Increases sense of physical beauty.

Queen Anne's Lace: Transforms sexuality into spirituality. Integrates lower with higher chakras.

Self-Heal: Promotes vital sense of self.

Snapdragon: Helps develop strong libido.

Sticky Monkey Flower: Helps express sexual feelings.

Yarrow: When taken with Echinacea and arnica, protects against harmful environmental influences.

FLOWER ESSENCE RECIPE

Note: Since the proper formula in flower essence recipes varies from woman to woman, I include only one here, a recipe I've used successfully with hundreds of women. If you want to experiment with additional recipes on your own, or with the help of a practitioner, I recommend using a good reference book. To my mind, the best is *Flower Essence Repertory: A Comprehensive Guide to North American and English Flower Essences for Emotional and Spiritual Well-Being,* by Patricia Kaminski and Richard Katz (published by the Flower Essence Society, P.O. Box 459, Nevada City, CA 95959; phone: 1-800-548-0075; fax: 916-265-6467).

SEXUAL VITALITY REJUVENATOR

1 oz. distilled water
2 drops brandy (preservative)
2 drops self-heal flower essence
2 drops hibiscus flower essence
2 drops crab apple flower essence

Mix and take two to four drops under tongue four times a day. Avoid eating any food within fifteen minutes before or after.

TEN COOKING HERBS
THAT IGNITE METABOLISM

Black peppercorns
Cardamom
Cayenne pepper
Cinnamon
Coriander
Cumin
Fennel
Garlic
Ginger
Turmeric

$\mathcal{H}$ERBS FOR SEXUAL HEALTH

Chaste Tree (VITEX): Nourishes the mucous membranes. Promotes progesterone.

Dandelion: Mover of blood and lymph. Regulates sex hormones.

Don Quai: Called "female ginseng." Regulates hormones.

Ginger: Regulates the eicosanoids, which balance metabolism.

Ginkgo: Stimulates blood flow to brain and extremities.

Gotu Kola: Most important rejuvenative herb in Ayurvedic medicine. Strengthens adrenals and purifies blood.

Licorice: Contains estriol and isoflavone, which act as rejuvenators of the endocrine system.

Milk Thistle: Strengthens liver and protects against environmental toxins.

Oat Straw: "Avena sative": Nourishes nervous and endocrine systems. Makes a great "love potion."

Siberian Ginseng: Rejuvenates adrenals and nervous system.

St. John's Wort: Mood elevator. Relieves depression and anxiety.

Turmeric: Regulates hormone function and promotes proper metabolism.

Wild Yam: Good source of zinc.

*N*UTRIENTS FOR SEXUALITY

Vitamin A: Antioxidant. Restores decreased thyroid levels.

B-complex: Contributes to production of sex hormones and to thyroid function.

Beta-carotene: Lubricates vagina. Increases progesterone levels.

Bioflavonoids: Supports cell membranes. Required by ovaries.

Vitamin C: Antioxidant. Strengthens cell walls and enhances activity of enzyme pathways. Required for progesterone secretion.

Calcium: Benefits nervous system and healthy bone function.

Vitamin E: Feeds pituitary and thyroid glands. Lubricates vagina. Prevents oxidation of essential fatty acids.

Magnesium: Activates enzymes to metabolize amino acids and promotes utilization of other vitamins in maintaining acid/base balance.

Selenium: Antioxidant. Helps protect body from environmental toxins. Good for thyroid, which affects libido.

Zinc: Vital for proper functioning of sex glands. Good for thyroid function and increased sex drive.

ᏔᎾOMEN'S APHRODISIACS

Remember: The best aphrodisiac is the mind.

Asparagus	Garlic
Cloves	Ginseng
Damiana	Hibiscus
Don quai	Onions
Fenugreek	Wild yams
Fo-ti	

WOMEN'S DAILY SEXUAL TONIC

$^1/_2$ tsp. licorice root
$^1/_2$ tsp. cardamom seeds
1 slice fresh ginger
Dash of cinnamon

Mix in one quart boiling water. Let steep for one to two minutes, then strain and ingest.

$\mathcal{S}$UGGESTED READING

Chia, Mantak, and Maneewan Chia. *Healing Love Through the Tao: Cultivating Female Sexual Energy.* Huntington, N.Y.: Healing Tao Books, 1986.

Colbin, Annemarie. *Food and Healing.* New York: Ballantine Books, 1986.

Frawley, David. *Ayurvedic Healing: A Comprehensive Guide.* Salt Lake City, Utah: Passage Press, 1989.

Frawley, David, and Lad Vascant. *The Yoga of Herbs: An Ayurvedic Guide to Herbal Medicine.* Twin Lakes, Wisc.: Lotus Light, 1986.

Golan, Ralph. *Optimal Wellness.* New York: Ballantine Books, 1995.

Johari, Harish. *Breath, Mind and Consciousness.* Rochester, N.Y.: Destine Books, 1989.

Kaminski, Patricia, and Richard Katz. *Flower Essence Repertory: A Comprehensive Guide to North American and English Flower Essences for Emotional and Spiritual Well-Being.* Nevada City, Calif.: The Flower Essence Society, 1994.

Lad, Vascant. *Ayurveda: The Science of Self-Healing.* Twin Lakes, Wisc.: Lotus Press, 1984.

Neurenberger, Philip. *The Quest for Personal Power: Transforming Stress into Strength*. New York: G. P. Putnam, 1996.

Northrup, Christiane. *Women's Bodies, Women's Wisdom: Creating Physical and Emotional Health and Healing*. New York: Bantam Books, 1995.

Pizzorne, Joseph. *Total Wellness*. Rocklin, Calif.: Prima Publishing, 1996.

Rechtschaffen, Stephan. *TimeShifting*. New York: Doubleday, 1996.

Reid, Daniel. *The Complete Book of Chinese Health and Healing*. Boston, Mass.: Shambala, 1995.

Shaw, Miranda. *Passionate Enlightenment: Women in Tantric Buddhism*. Princeton, N.J.: Princeton University Press, 1994.

Svoboda, Robert. *Prakruti: Your Ayurvedic Constitution*. Albuquerque, N.M.: Geocom, 1988.

Svoboda, Robert, and Arnie Lade. *Tao and Dharma*. Twin Lakes, Wisc.: Lotus Press, 1995.

Tisserand, Robert B. *The Art of Aromatherapy*. Rochester, Vt.: Healing Arts Press, 1977.

Tyler, Varro E. *Herbs of Choice: The Therapeutic Use of Phytomedicinals*. Binghamton, N.Y.: Hawthorn Press, 1994.

Weed, Susan. *Menopausal Years: The Wise Woman Way*. Woodstock, N.Y.: Ash Tree Publishing, 1992.

$\mathcal{I}$ NDEX

ABOUT THE AUTHOR

Dr. Susan Taylor received her Ph.D. in nutritional biochemistry from Case Western Reserve University School of Medicine and her M.S. in human nutrition from Columbia University. A medical consultant to physicians, businesses, and individual clients, Dr. Taylor lectures and gives workshops nationally. Information on Dr. Taylor's seminars, lectures, workshops, and classes is available by calling (303) 786-9652 or visiting her Web site: www.drsusantaylor.com.